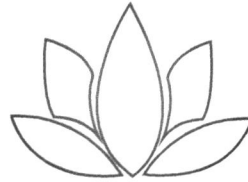

CHAIR YOGA FOR SENIORS 3 IN 1 THE COMPLETE COLLECTION

Mobility and Balance + Strength Training + Pain Management | Quick and Easy Chair Exercises For Beginners

J.C. Harrison

Gran Publications

Legal Notice

Disclaimer

This publication is provided "as is" without warranty of any kind, expressed or implied, including but not limited to warranties of performance, merchantability, fitness for a particular purpose, accuracy, omissions, completeness, currentness, or delays. The information in this book is for educational and entertainment purposes only. Efforts have been made to ensure that the content herein is accurate and up to date; however, the author and publisher make no guarantees concerning the accuracy or applicability of any content. Readers should independently verify any information within this book.

The content of this book is not intended to be a substitute for professional advice. Should you require advice in a specific field, consult with a licensed professional who is qualified to provide such counsel. The author and publisher shall not be liable for any damages arising from the use, misuse, or interpretation of the information contained herein. The reader assumes full responsibility for their actions and the consequences thereof.

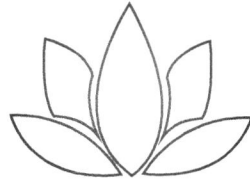

CONTENTS

PART I - CHAIR YOGA FOR MOBILITY & BALANCE

CHAPTER 4
CHAIR YOGA FOR UPPER BODY PAIN AND SHOULDER PAIN   116

CHAPTER 5
CHAIR YOGA FOR COMBATING MUSCLE STIFFNESS AND PAIN   128

CHAPTER 6
YOUR FLEXIBLE CHAIR YOGA ROUTINE FOR PAIN RELIEF   138

CONCLUSION   140

PART III - CHAIR YOGA FOR STRENGTH

CHAPTER 4
CHAIR YOGA FOR LOWER BODY STRENGTH   **180**

CHAPTER 5
CHAIR YOGA FOR BALANCE AND COORDINATION   **190**

CHAPTER 6
CHAIR YOGA FOR FLEXIBILITY AND MOBILITY   **200**

CHAPTER 7
CHAIR YOGA FOR POSTURE AND ALIGNMENT
210

CHAPTER 8
YOUR FLEXIBLE CHAIR YOGA ROUTINE FOR STRENGTH
220

CONCLUSION
222

REFERENCES
224

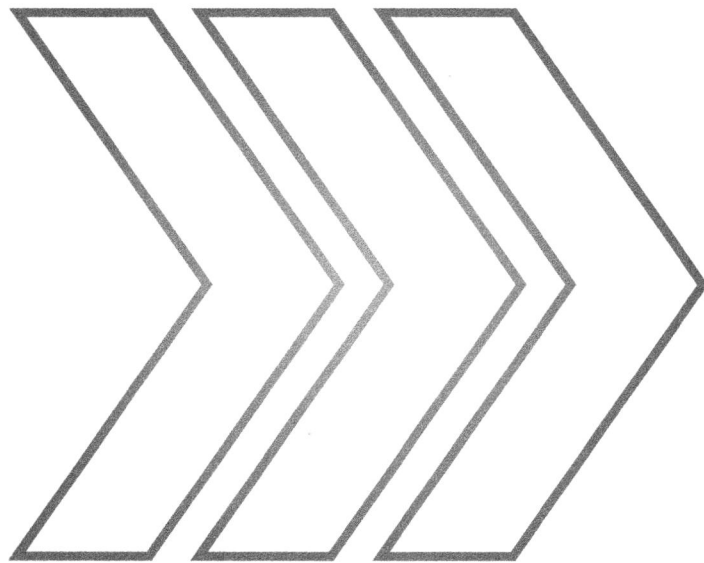

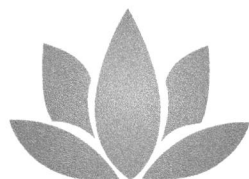

PART I
CHAIR YOGA
FOR MOBILITY & BALANCE

Gentle Seated Exercises for Better Flexibility, Increased Strength, Improved Posture, Faster Weight Loss and Pain Relief in Senior's Quick and Easy Workouts.

J.C. Harrison

Gran Publications

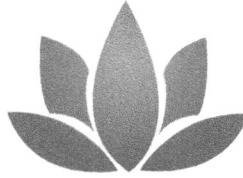

INTRODUCTION

Imagine the frustration of watching the world around you move with ease while you struggle to keep up. For many seniors, the simplest tasks become monumental challenges. The joy of kneeling down to tend to a garden, walking through the park, or playing with your grandchildren fades into a memory as mobility issues take hold. Everyday activities that once brought so much joy and freedom now seem daunting and, at times, impossible. This sense of loss can lead to feelings of isolation and helplessness as if the world is slipping away bit by bit. You might miss out on family gatherings, skip outings with friends, or feel unable to participate in your favorite hobbies. These moments can be incredibly disheartening, but there is a gentle and effective solution that can help.

My name is JC Harrison, and I've dedicated my life to helping seniors reclaim their mobility, independence, and joy through chair yoga. Inspired by my own mother's journey to maintain her fitness and health as she grew older, I created a comprehensive chair yoga program tailored specifically for seniors. With years of experience in senior fitness and wellness, I help seniors become pain-free, increase their mobility, and regain their independence, all from the comfort of their chair!

My mission is simple: help as many moms, dads, grandpas, and grandmas play with their grandkids and live their golden years the way they always wanted. Through my books and our supportive online community, I aim to empower seniors to take control of their health and well-being. I believe that everyone, regardless of age or physical limitations, deserves to live a life full of vitality and happiness. My mission is to provide you with the tools and guidance needed to overcome mobility issues and rediscover the activities you love. Whether you're dealing with chronic pain, or stiffness, or simply looking for a way to stay active, I'm here to help you every step of the way.

Chair Yoga can do wonders for you and before we dive into the how, why and what it is all about, I want to share three quick stories from real members in our community with you.

Many members of our supportive community have shared their inspiring journeys of transformation through chair yoga. Consider Jane, a vibrant woman in her late seventies who always took pride in her active lifestyle. Gardening was her passion, and she spent hours cultivating her little piece of paradise. However, as the years passed, Jane began to notice a creeping stiffness in her joints. The once-simple act of kneeling to plant flowers became an ordeal, and soon, she found herself unable to maintain her beloved garden. Jane shared her story in our Facebook group, describing the pain and frustration that had become constant companions in her life. But then, Jane discovered chair yoga. With regular practice, she regained her flexibility and strength, allowing her to return to her cherished gardening with newfound ease and joy.

Another inspiring story comes from Tom, an avid photographer who loved capturing nature's beauty. For years, Tom would venture into the woods with his camera, photographing birds and wildlife. However, as his mobility declined, so did his ability to navigate the uneven terrain of his favorite trails. The walks that once filled him with joy and creativity became strenuous and painful, forcing him to give up his beloved hobby. Tom felt a profound sense of loss, not just for the physical activity, but for the creative outlet that brought him so much happiness. After joining our chair yoga program, Tom gradually regained his strength and flexibility. He shared in our community how he was able to return to his nature walks, camera in hand, capturing the moments that he thought were lost forever.

And then there's Mary, who faced the daily challenge of getting up from her favorite chair. Each attempt to stand felt like an insurmountable task, leaving her feeling defeated and dependent on others. Mary's frustration and sense of loss were echoed by many seniors in our group. However, with regular chair yoga practice, Mary gradually built up the strength in her legs and core. Today, she stands up with ease and moves around her home confidently. Mary now enjoys a renewed sense of accomplishment and independence that she once thought was beyond her reach.

Now, let's talk about why you should care about chair yoga. This isn't just another exercise fad. Chair yoga offers real, tangible benefits that can transform your daily life. Imagine waking up each morning with more ease and less stiffness, moving through your day with renewed confidence and vitality. Chair yoga is about making those frustrating limitations a thing of the past and reclaiming the freedom to enjoy life fully.

Picture yourself feeling more flexible and agile, able to reach for that top shelf or bend down to pick something up without hesitation. Envision having the strength to move around your home with ease, tackling daily chores and activities without the constant fear of falling. Chair yoga helps enhance your balance and coordination, making you steadier on your feet and reducing the risk of falls.

Consider the relief of living with less pain. Many seniors report significant reductions in chronic pain after incorporating chair yoga into their routine. This newfound comfort allows you to participate in activities you love, like gardening, walking in the park, or spending quality time with your grandchildren, without being held back by discomfort.

Think about the improvement in your overall well-being. With better circulation, your body feels more energized and alive. Improved posture means standing and sitting tall, exuding confidence and ease. The mindful breathing and stretching exercises help release muscle tension, leaving you feeling more relaxed and at peace.

Imagine the joy of regaining the independence you thought was lost. Simple tasks, like standing up from a chair or climbing a few stairs, become achievable goals, bringing a sense of accomplishment and pride. The gentle movements of chair yoga encourage the production of synovial fluid, which keeps your joints lubricated and functioning smoothly, enhancing your mobility and reducing the risk of injuries.

By starting at your own pace and gradually increasing the intensity, chair yoga allows your body to adapt and strengthen over time. This gradual progression ensures that you build your capabilities safely and effectively, leading to a more active and fulfilling lifestyle.

Chair yoga isn't just about physical movement; it's about transforming your daily experiences and reclaiming the joy and freedom to live your golden years to the fullest.

Here is what you can expect

In this book, you'll find a comprehensive guide to chair yoga designed specifically for seniors, focusing on enhancing mobility and overall well-being. We'll start with the basics, helping you set up a comfortable and safe space for your practice. From there, we'll explore warm-up exercises to prepare your body for more intensive stretches and movements.

We'll delve into techniques to enhance joint flexibility and muscle strengthening, ensuring your body stays limber and strong. You'll learn exercises to improve your balance and coordination, reducing the risk of falls and enhancing your stability. We'll cover methods to alleviate chronic pain, helping you move more comfortably through your day.

As we progress, we'll focus on improving circulation to keep your body energized and improving posture to help you stand and sit tall with confidence. You'll discover ways to reduce muscle tension through stretching and mindful breathing, promoting relaxation and peace. We'll also explore exercises to increase joint lubrication, keep your joints functioning smoothly, and enhance muscle elasticity to reduce the risk of injury.

Finally, we'll discuss the gradual progression of movement exercises, starting at your own pace and increasing intensity as your body adapts and strengthens. By the end of this book, you'll have a complete toolkit of chair yoga exercises designed to help you reclaim your mobility, reduce pain, and live a more active and fulfilling life

By embracing chair yoga as a daily practice, you are choosing to prioritize your health and well-being, taking proactive steps to alleviate discomfort and enhance your quality of life. Through dedication and consistency, you have the power to transform how you experience pain and cultivate a sense of balance and harmony within your body and mind.

Remember, every small step you take towards improving your mobility counts. Chair yoga is not just about physical movement; it's about reclaiming your independence and rediscovering the joys of daily activities. Let this book be your guide on this empowering journey towards better mobility and a more fulfilling life. This is your chance to take control and show those mobility issues who's boss.

You've got this, and I'm here to help you every step of the way.

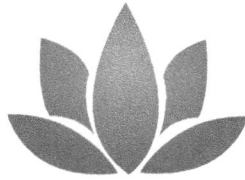

CHAPTER 1
CHAIR YOGA FOR
MOBILITY AND BALANCE

WHAT IS CHAIR YOGA?

Chair yoga is your gateway to fitness, no matter your age or mobility level. Designed with seniors in mind, it adapts traditional yoga poses to be performed while seated or using a chair for support. This isn't about watering down yoga; it's about making it work for you. Chair yoga lets you reap all the benefits of yoga—flexibility, strength, balance—without the risk of injury or strain. It's perfect for those who find standing or floor-based poses challenging. By incorporating a chair, you can safely and effectively perform a wide range of poses, boosting your mobility and overall well-being. It's time to take charge of your health and feel the transformation!

Chair yoga is uniquely tailored to meet the needs of older adults, providing a safe and effective way to improve mobility and overall well-being. Regular practice can lead to numerous benefits:

» **Enhanced Joint Flexibility**: The gentle stretches in chair yoga help keep your joints limber and reduce stiffness, making everyday movements easier.

» **Muscle Strengthening**: Even mild resistance exercises can build muscle strength, offering better support for your joints and enhancing your ability to perform daily tasks.

» **Improved Balance and Coordination**: Chair yoga improves your stability and coordination, which is crucial for reducing the risk of falls and maintaining independence.

» **Pain Reduction**: Many seniors experience significant reductions in chronic pain, such as back pain or arthritis, through regular chair yoga practice.

» **Improved Circulation**: The movements in chair yoga encourage better blood flow throughout your body, which is essential for maintaining overall health and vitality.

» **Improved Posture**: Strengthening your core muscles and increasing your body awareness can lead to better posture, helping you stand and sit tall with confidence.

» **Reduced Muscle Tension**: The combination of stretching and mindful breathing in chair yoga helps release tension held in your muscles, promoting relaxation and reducing discomfort.

» **Increased Joint Lubrication**: Gentle movements stimulate the production of synovial fluid, which keeps your joints lubricated and functioning smoothly.

» **Better Muscle Elasticity**: Regular stretching enhances muscle elasticity, reducing the risk of injuries and making your body more resilient.

» **Gradual Progression of Movement Exercises**: Chair yoga allows you to start at your own pace and gradually increase the intensity as your body adapts and strengthens, ensuring a safe and effective progression.

By incorporating chair yoga into your routine, you can enjoy these benefits and experience a significant improvement in your quality of life, making daily activities more enjoyable and less challenging.

One of the best things about chair yoga is its gentle approach. It's a safe and accessible way for seniors to stay active, even if mobility is an issue. With smart modifications and the use of props, everyone can join in without worrying about injury. Chairs, blocks, and straps aren't just accessories; they're game-changers. These tools make poses more accessible and comfortable, helping you get the correct alignment and support. This means you maximize the benefits of every single exercise. It's all about making yoga work for you, no matter where you're starting from.

IMPORTANCE OF CHAIR YOGA FOR SENIOR HEALTH

Yoga isn't just exercise; it's a jump start for both your body and mind. For seniors, chair yoga paves the way to better mobility, less pain, and a higher quality of life. It boosts balance, flexibility, and posture, which are key to staying mobile as we age. The gentle stretches and strength-building moves in chair yoga keep your body in top shape, fighting off the decline that often comes with getting older.

But let's not forget the mental perks. Regular yoga practice slashes stress, sharpens focus, and brings a wave of calm. For seniors, this means better mental health and a brighter outlook on life. Plus, joining yoga classes, even online, builds a sense of community. Our supportive Facebook group (link at the back of the book) or local classes can help you beat isolation and connect with like-minded people.

Stick with yoga, and you'll add quality years to your life. By keeping your body and mind in check, you'll enjoy your golden years with more energy, independence, and vitality. It's all about living your best life, starting now.

HOW CHAIR YOGA WILL GET YOU MOVING AGAIN

Mobility is key to staying independent and enjoying life to the fullest. Chair yoga is a powerhouse tool, but it's just one part of a broader strategy to boost mobility.

Mobility issues can stem from conditions like arthritis, osteoporosis, strokes, hip and knee problems, chronic pain, balance disorders, muscle weakness, neuropathy, post-surgery recovery, obesity, respiratory issues, cognitive decline, and peripheral artery disease. Chair yoga tackles these head-on by improving joint flexibility, muscle strength, balance, pain management, circulation, posture, muscle tension, joint lubrication, and muscle elasticity. It's a gentle yet powerful way to enhance mobility, complementing traditional strategies perfectly.

For **arthritis sufferers**, chair yoga eases joint stiffness and cuts down inflammation with gentle stretches. The slow, controlled movements help maintain and even boost joint flexibility, making daily activities smoother and less painful.

If you're dealing with **osteoporosis**, chair yoga offers low-impact, weight-bearing exercises that strengthen bones and muscles safely, reducing the risk of fractures and improving bone density over time.

Stroke survivors can reap major benefits too. Chair yoga focuses on gentle, repetitive movements that help retrain the brain and body, enhancing coordination and strength on the affected side, and leading to better overall mobility and independence.

For those with **hip and knee issues**, especially post-replacement, chair yoga's low-impact exercises improve joint flexibility and muscle strength. This supports the joints, making walking and standing less painful and more stable.

For those battling **chronic pain**, chair yoga offers a holistic, effective way to manage it. Gentle stretching, strengthening exercises, and mindful breathing techniques work together to improve circulation and release muscle tension, alleviating pain naturally.

Balance disorders can be particularly challenging, but chair yoga targets stability through specific exercises that enhance balance and coordination. This reduces the risk of falls and helps you feel more secure in your movements.

Chair yoga's focus on **mindful movement and breathwork** also boosts circulation, ensuring blood flows freely throughout your body. This is vital for overall health, especially for those with conditions like peripheral artery disease or diabetes, which can impair circulation.

Enhancing posture through core-strengthening exercises, chair yoga helps alleviate strain on your back and other areas, promoting better alignment and reducing pain. Improved posture also leads to better balance and coordination, making everyday movements safer and more efficient.

Muscle tension is common among seniors, often worsened by stress and a sedentary lifestyle. Chair yoga's gentle stretches and relaxation techniques help release this tension, leading to greater comfort and relaxation.

The production of **synovial fluid** is stimulated through chair yoga's gentle, repetitive movements, keeping joints lubricated and functioning smoothly. This reduces friction and wear within the joints, enhancing mobility and reducing pain.

Regular chair yoga practice also improves **muscle elasticity**, making muscles more resilient and less prone to injury. This allows for a broader range of motion and greater flexibility, which is essential for maintaining mobility and independence as we age.

In summary, chair yoga provides a comprehensive, gentle approach to addressing the root causes of mobility issues. It complements traditional treatments and strategies, offering a safe and effective way to enhance mobility, reduce pain, and improve the overall quality of life for seniors. By incorporating chair yoga into your routine, you're taking proactive steps towards better health and greater independence.

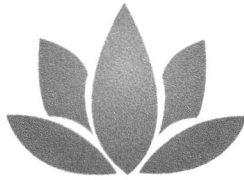

CHAPTER 2
CREATING A SERENE SPACE FOR YOUR CHAIR YOGA ROUTINE

Creating a space that invites tranquility and mindfulness is the first step in preparing for chair yoga. A serene environment not only sets the tone for your practice but also contributes to the effectiveness of each session. The right atmosphere fosters peace and minimizes distractions, making it easier to focus on movements and breathing. By taking the time to organize and beautify your yoga area, you lay the groundwork for a rewarding and focused exercise routine.

This chapter will guide you through the process of selecting the ideal chair that offers both stability and comfort for your yoga practice. You'll learn about adjusting your space to ensure it's safe and conducive to mindful movement, with tips on choosing chairs with proper support and how to personalize your seating arrangement. Additionally, the discussion extends to creating a calm and clutter-free environment, using lighting and personal touches to enhance relaxation. With these insights, you'll be well-prepared to embark on a fulfilling journey of chair yoga, enriching both your physical and mental well-being.

CHOOSING THE RIGHT CHAIR

Selecting the right chair is crucial for safety and comfort. Here's what you need to know:

» **Height and Stability**: Your feet should be flat on the ground to maintain balance. Measure the distance from the floor to your knees while seated; this should match the chair height. Avoid chairs with wheels or swivel mechanisms. Metal or wooden chairs are usually more stable than plastic ones.

» **Back Support**: A chair with a sturdy backrest helps maintain proper spinal alignment. Consider chairs with lumbar support or add a cushion behind your lower back if needed.

» **Armrests and Cushioning**: Choose a chair without armrests or one that is wide enough to leave several inches of space between your body and the armrests, so you can have plenty of room for your movements. Cushioned seats prevent pressure points, especially important for those with sensitive joints or arthritis. Use thick seat pads or cushions if your chair lacks padding.

CREATING A PEACEFUL SPACE

A clutter-free environment fosters focus and relaxation. Here's how to create one:

» **Clear Clutter**: Remove unnecessary items from your yoga area. Use shelves or baskets to organize essentials.

» **Lighting**: Soft, natural light creates a calming atmosphere. Practice near a window if possible, or use warm-toned light bulbs to mimic natural daylight.

» **Relaxing Elements**: Add plants, calming artwork, and elements like tabletop fountains or essential oil diffusers to enhance relaxation.

» **Personal Touches**: Include cherished items like family photos or favorite books. Use calming scents like lavender or eucalyptus to promote relaxation.

MINDFUL BREATHING AND TECHNIQUES TO CENTER YOUR THOUGHTS

Getting your mind in the right place is just as crucial as the physical aspects of chair yoga. Setting positive intentions and preparing mentally helps you get the most out of your practice by creating a distraction-free zone filled with anticipation for healing. Mindfulness and positive affirmations turn your physical exercise into a holistic experience that nurtures both body and spirit. Here are some of my favorite ones to help get started with. You don't need to use all of them, just choose the ones you enjoy the most and use them.

Start with mindful breathing techniques to calm your mind before chair yoga.

Diaphragmatic Breathing

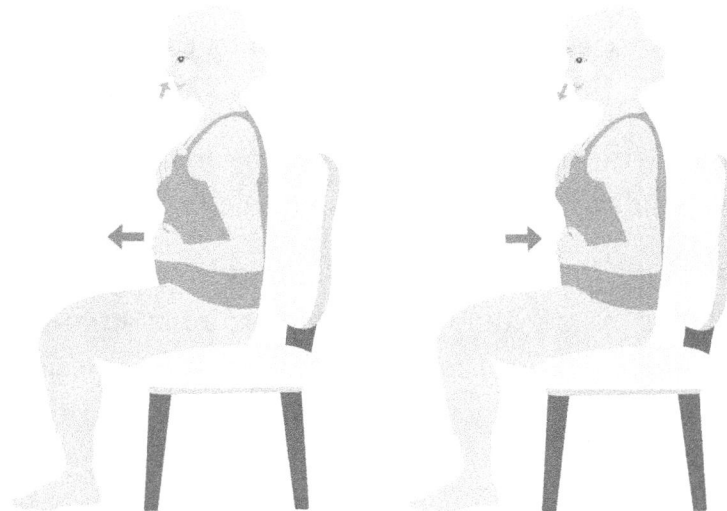

A simple yet powerful exercise, here's how to practice it:
1. Sit comfortably.
2. Place one hand on your chest and the other on your abdomen.
3. Take slow, deep breaths.
4. Focus on making your abdomen rise more than your chest.
5. Exhale slowly.
6. Repeat to reduce anxiety and promote relaxation.

Box Breathing

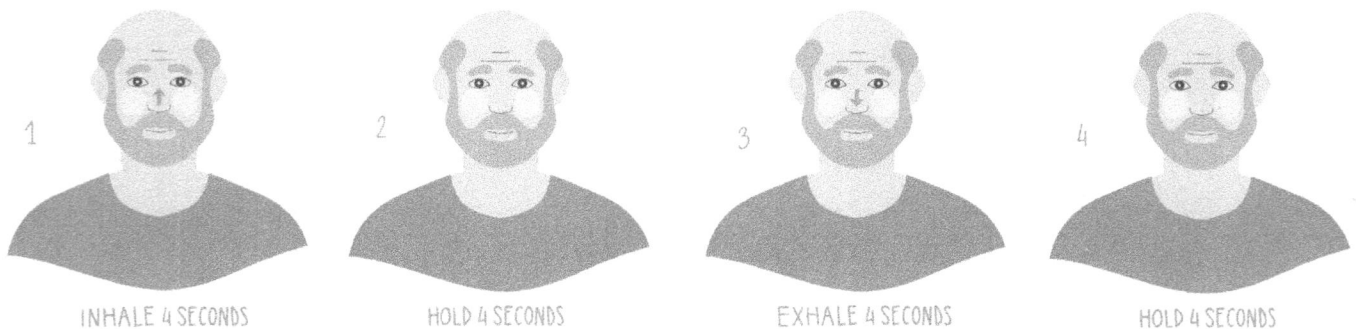

INHALE 4 SECONDS   HOLD 4 SECONDS   EXHALE 4 SECONDS   HOLD 4 SECONDS

This exercise can further refine your practice. The structured pattern not only ensures a regular breathing rhythm but also helps detach your mind from stressful thoughts, providing a sense of control and peace. Here's how to do it:

1. Sit comfortably.
2. Inhale deeply for a count of four.
3. Hold for a count of four.
4. Exhale slowly for a count of four.
5. Repeat this pattern to ensure a regular breathing rhythm and detach from stressful thoughts.

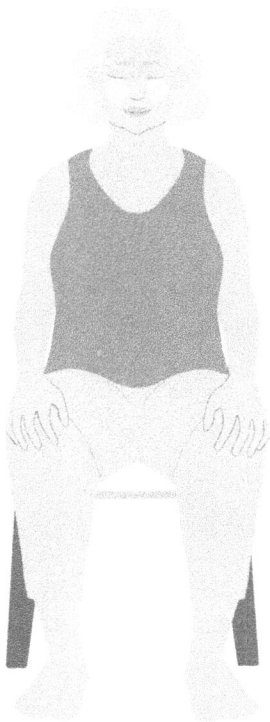

Breath Awareness

Another technique to enhance focus, follow these steps to put it in practice:

1. Sit comfortably with your spine straight and hands resting on your knees.
2. Close your eyes and focus solely on the sensation of air moving in and out.
3. If your mind wanders, gently bring your focus back to your breath.

Centering your thoughts is crucial for effective mental preparation in chair yoga. Grounding techniques, such as focusing on the present moment, are invaluable. Mindfulness practices, like paying attention to your body's sensations or the sounds around you, help anchor your mind in the "now." This reduces stress and ensures that your mind and body move in harmony, enhancing the overall effectiveness of your yoga practice. Here are some techniques you can try to center your thoughts.

Body Scanning

One powerful way to ground yourself is through Body Scanning.
1. Start at the top of your head and work your way down to your toes.
2. Note any areas of tension or discomfort without trying to change them.
3. Bring awareness to each part of your body.
4. Focus on a single word or phrase, such as "peace" or "calm," and repeat it silently to yourself while breathing deeply.

Guided Imagery

Guided imagery is also a potent tool for centering thoughts. Guided imagery helps center your thoughts and cultivate a serene mindset:
1. Visualize a tranquil scene, such as a beach or forest.
2. Imagine yourself in that setting.
3. Focus on the sensory details—sights, sounds, and smells.
4. Let this imagery create a profound sense of relaxation and presence.

Visualizing a Pain-Free State

Visualizing a pain-free state can dramatically enhance the benefits of chair yoga. Use guided imagery to envision yourself free from discomfort, fostering a more optimistic outlook towards the practice. The brain's relationship with pain is complex, and visualization can play a significant role in altering pain perception.
1. Find a comfortable seated position.
2. Close your eyes and take several deep breaths to center yourself.
3. Imagine a warm, healing light surrounding the area of discomfort.
4. Picture this light slowly melting away the pain, leaving behind a sensation of relief and comfort.

In addition to pain-specific visualization, imagine yourself performing chair yoga poses effortlessly. Visualize the ease with which you move and the joy you feel in each stretch. This mental rehearsal can prepare your body to replicate those smooth motions in real life, enhancing your practice's fluidity and enjoyment. Over time, consistent visualization can lead to actual improvements in mobility and pain levels.

Embracing a Positive Mindset

Embracing a positive mindset is essential to maximize the benefits of chair yoga. It's easy to focus on limitations, especially when dealing with chronic pain or reduced mobility. However, cultivating a mindset that sees possibilities rather than restrictions can transform your practice and overall well-being. Positivity isn't about ignoring pain or discomfort; it's about recognizing your body's efforts and celebrating small victories.

One strategy to maintain a positive outlook is through Affirmations. These are positive statements that you repeat to yourself to challenge and overcome negative thoughts. For example, phrases like "I am strong," "I am capable," or "I am improving every day" can gradually shift your mindset from what you can't do to what you can achieve. Incorporating these affirmations at the beginning and end of your chair yoga sessions can reinforce your commitment to positive change.

Remember, your chair yoga practice is a journey. Adjust your environment and mental practices to suit your needs, and prioritize safety and comfort. These thoughtful preparations lead to regular, enjoyable yoga sessions, contributing to long-term well-being.

In closing, integrating a well-chosen chair, a serene space, and dedicated mental preparation paves the way for a rewarding chair yoga practice that nurtures both body and mind. Cherish the moments of peace and relaxation, and let your chair yoga practice become a cornerstone of your well-being journey.

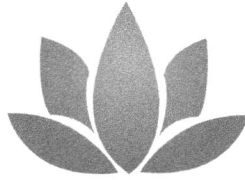

CHAPTER 3
THE WARM-UP ADVANTAGE: WHY IT'S ESSENTIAL FOR YOUR WORKOUT

Alright, folks! Warming up and stretching are essential parts of any exercise routine, especially for seniors. These activities prepare your body for the work ahead and help keep you injury-free. Think of warm-ups as the ignition switch that gets your engine running, and stretching as the maintenance that keeps everything smooth and functional.

Warm-ups are exercises designed to gradually increase your heart rate and blood flow to muscles. They prime your body for the activity that's about to come. Different types of warm-ups include cardiovascular exercises like brisk walking and dynamic stretches that get your muscles moving.

TYPES OF WARM-UP EXERCISES

» **Cardiovascular Warm-Ups:** Activities like brisk walking or marching in place. They get your heart pumping and muscles warmed up.

» **Dynamic Stretches:** Movements that take your muscles through a full range of motion, like gentle leg swings or arm circles.

BENEFITS OF WARM-UPS

Incorporating warm-ups into your routine helps set the stage for a more effective and safe chair yoga practice. First and foremost, warm-ups increase muscle temperature, which makes your muscles more flexible and efficient. Think of it like warming up your car on a cold morning; your body performs better when it's properly warmed up.

Additionally, warm-ups enhance oxygen delivery to your muscles. This improvement in oxygen flow boosts your endurance, allowing you to sustain your yoga poses longer and with better form. It's like giving your muscles a breath of fresh air, ensuring they're ready to work hard and recover quickly.

Moreover, warm-ups prime your nervous system for peak performance. By engaging in gentle movements before diving into your main routine, you signal to your body that it's time to get active. This readiness translates to smoother, more coordinated movements and greater overall effectiveness in your chair yoga session.

Finally, warm-ups play a crucial role in reducing the risk of injuries. By gradually preparing your muscles and joints for the activity ahead, you minimize the chances of strains, sprains, and other injuries. It's all about setting the foundation for a safe, productive, and enjoyable chair yoga practice.

In short, making warm-ups a non-negotiable part of your routine can significantly enhance your chair yoga experience, leading to better flexibility, endurance, performance, and injury prevention.

DESIGNING AN EFFECTIVE WARM-UP ROUTINE

» General Warm-Up

Starting with a light cardiovascular activity to increase your heart rate is especially important for seniors dealing with pain issues. This phase helps to get your blood flowing and raise your body temperature, which can alleviate stiffness and discomfort. Engaging in activities like brisk walking or gentle cycling at a low intensity can ease joint pain and improve mobility. This gradual increase in heart rate and circulation ensures that your muscles are ready for more intense activity, reducing the likelihood of aggravating existing pain.

» Dynamic Stretching

Incorporating dynamic stretching into your warm-up is vital for improving flexibility and managing pain. Unlike static stretching, dynamic stretches involve continuous movement, which helps to lubricate the joints and increase their range of motion. Exercises like leg swings, arm circles, and torso twists gently stretch your muscles, enhancing their elasticity and reducing stiffness. For seniors, this can mean less pain and better mobility throughout the day, as dynamic stretching prepares the body for the demands of exercise while minimizing the risk of injury.

» Activity-Specific Warm-Up

Performing exercises that mimic the movements of your workout is crucial for seniors experiencing pain. This type of warm-up ensures that your muscles and joints are adequately prepared for specific activities, which can help to prevent flare-ups of pain. For example, if you're planning to walk or run, incorporating movements like high knees or butt kicks can activate the relevant muscle groups and improve coordination. For weightlifting or resistance exercises, practice movements that replicate the lifts you'll be performing to reduce strain on your joints and muscles.

» For Aerobic Workouts

When preparing for aerobic workouts, seniors should begin with a 5-minute brisk walk. This activity is gentle on the joints while effectively increasing your heart rate and promoting blood flow. Follow up with dynamic stretches such as knee lifts and arm swings. Knee lifts target your hip flexors and lower body, areas often affected by pain, while arm swings engage your shoulders and upper body. These movements help to loosen up your muscles, reducing stiffness and making aerobic exercise more comfortable.

CUSTOMIZING YOUR WARM-UP

Everyone's needs are different, so it's important to customize your warm-up by considering the following:

» **Fitness Level:** If you're a beginner, you might need a longer warm-up to adequately prepare your body for exercise.

» **Type of Workout:** Tailor your warm-up to match the specific activities you'll be doing. For example, a warm-up for a cardio session will look different from one for strength training.

» **Personal Preferences**: Include movements that you enjoy and that make you feel ready for your workout. This can help make your warm-up more effective and enjoyable.

IMPORTANCE OF STRETCHING

Regular stretching offers numerous benefits that can enhance your overall well-being. It can significantly improve flexibility and range of motion, allowing you to move more freely and perform daily activities with ease. Additionally, stretching enhances muscular coordination, ensuring that your muscles work together efficiently during movement.

Stretching also increases blood flow to your muscles, which helps to deliver essential nutrients and oxygen, promoting muscle health and recovery. Maintaining proper posture is another key benefit of regular stretching, as it helps to align your body correctly and reduce the risk of postural issues.

Moreover, stretching can reduce muscle tension and soreness, making you feel more relaxed and comfortable after workouts or long periods of inactivity.

GUIDELINES FOR SAFE STRETCHING

To stretch safely and effectively, it's important to follow some essential guidelines:

» **Warm Up First**: Always warm up before stretching. Stretching cold muscles can lead to injuries, so engage in light cardiovascular activity to get your blood flowing.

» **Avoid Bouncing**: Use slow, steady movements when stretching. Bouncing can cause muscle strain and lead to injuries.

» **Hold Each Stretch**: Aim to hold each stretch for 15-30 seconds, remembering to stretch both sides equally. Stretching should be done without discomfort; you should feel a gentle pull but not pain.

» **Breathe**: Remember to breathe deeply during your stretches. Don't hold your breath; instead, inhale and exhale deeply to help your muscles relax and maximize the benefits of stretching.

Upper Body Stretches

» **Shoulder Stretch**: Bring your right arm across your body, using your left hand to press it gently towards your chest. Switch arms after a few breaths.

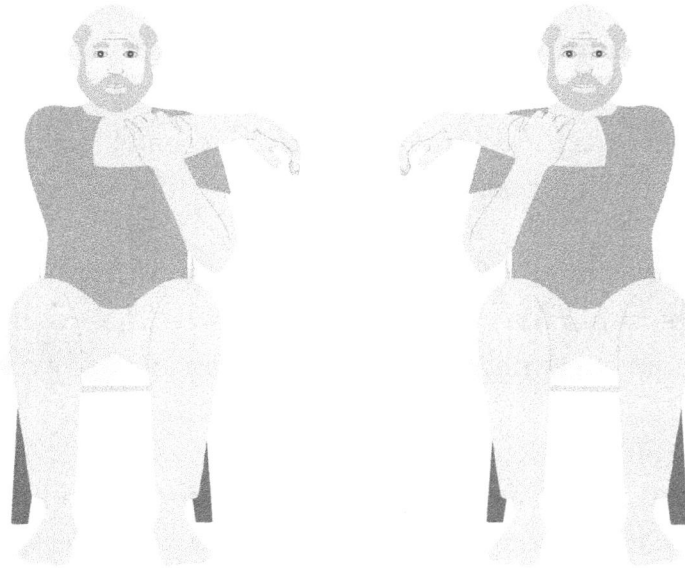

» **Torso Twists**: Sit upright with your feet flat on the floor. Place your hands on your knees. Gently twist your torso to the right, then to the left, warming up the spine.

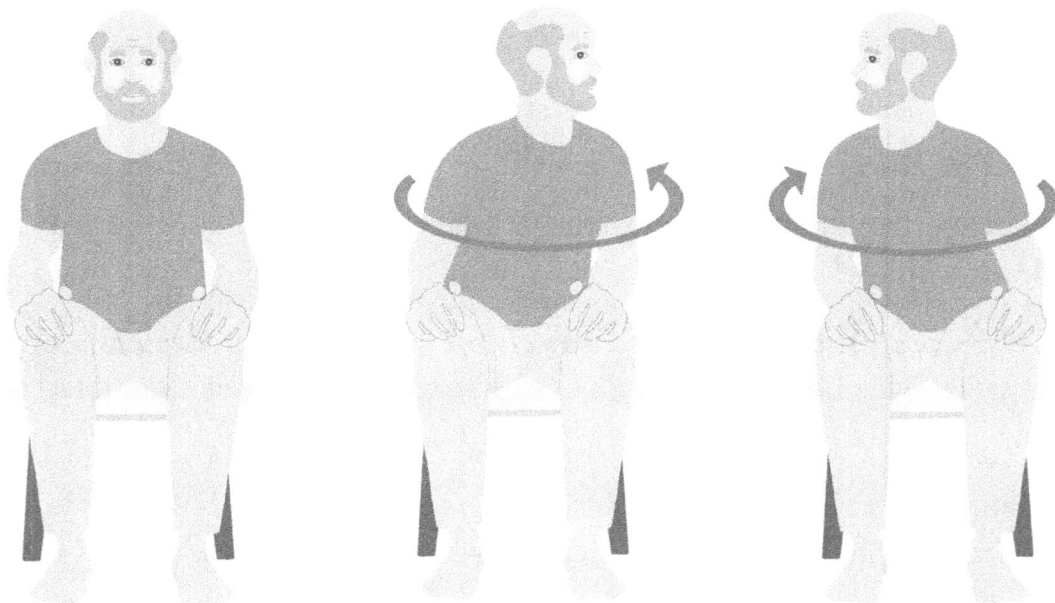

Lower Body Stretches

» **Toe and Heel Lifts**: With your feet flat on the floor, lift your toes while keeping your heels down, then lift your heels while keeping your toes down. This exercise warms up the feet and calves.

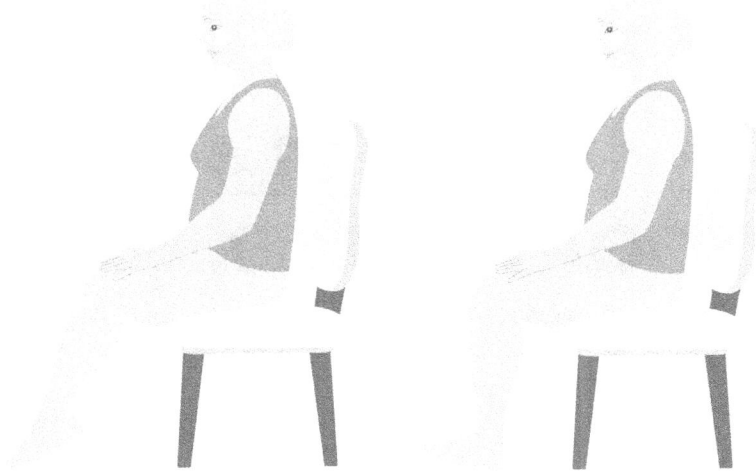

» **Ankle and Wrist Rotations**: Rotate your wrists and ankles slowly in both directions. This helps to loosen the joints and improve circulation.

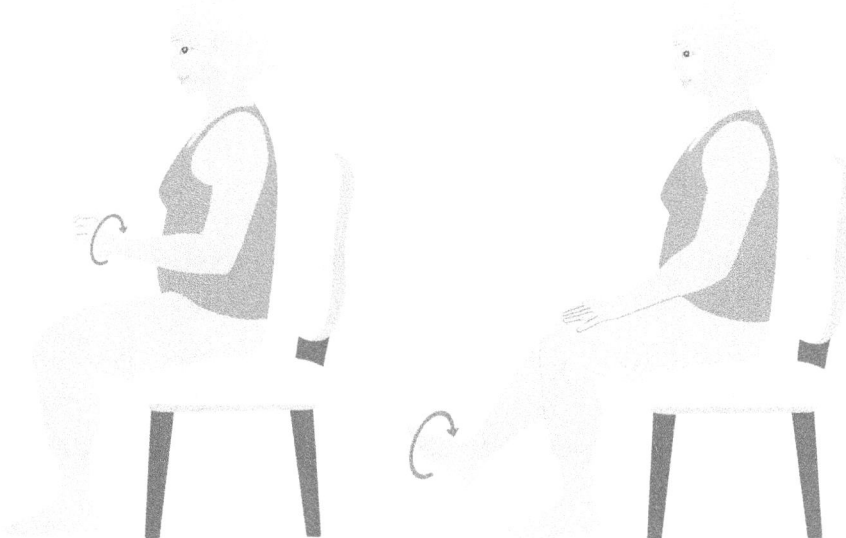

Wrapping it up, warm-ups and stretching are crucial for any workout regimen, especially for seniors. They prepare your body, enhance performance, and prevent injuries. Incorporate these practices into your routine to ensure you're always ready to give it your best. Stay consistent, listen to your body, and keep pushing your limits safely!

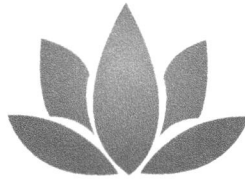

CHAPTER 4
CHAIR YOGA FOR FLEXIBILITY AND JOINT HEALTH

Alright, let's get real about what happens to our bodies as we age. Our joints and muscles can become stiff, limiting flexibility and reducing mobility. This stiffness can turn simple daily tasks like reaching, bending, and even walking into challenging feats. But guess what? You don't have to settle for that. Chair yoga is here to help you regain flexibility and improve your joint health without putting yourself at risk.

The poses selected for this chapter are tailor-picked to enhance your flexibility and joint health. Each one has been chosen for its effectiveness in targeting the areas most commonly affected by stiffness and limited mobility. These movements are not only easy on the body but also incredibly effective in improving joint function and overall flexibility. By incorporating these exercises into your daily routine, you can gradually increase your range of motion and alleviate the stiffness that often comes with aging. These movements don't just target specific areas of stiffness; they promote overall well-being. Improved joint health and flexibility can lead to a more active, independent, and fulfilling lifestyle. So, grab your chair and let's get started on this journey to a more flexible, mobile you.

Seated Spinal Twist

Helps with:	
» **Enhanced joint flexibility** This pose gently stretches and rotates the spine, improving flexibility in the vertebrae and surrounding joints.	» **Pain reduction** Twisting the spine helps relieve tension in the lower back and shoulders, reducing pain.
» **Improved posture** It encourages proper alignment of the spine, helping to improve overall posture.	» **Reduced muscle tension** The twisting motion helps release tightness in the back and shoulder muscles.

Safety Precautions:

- Twist gently, avoiding any forceful movements.
- If you have a spine condition, consult a healthcare professional first.

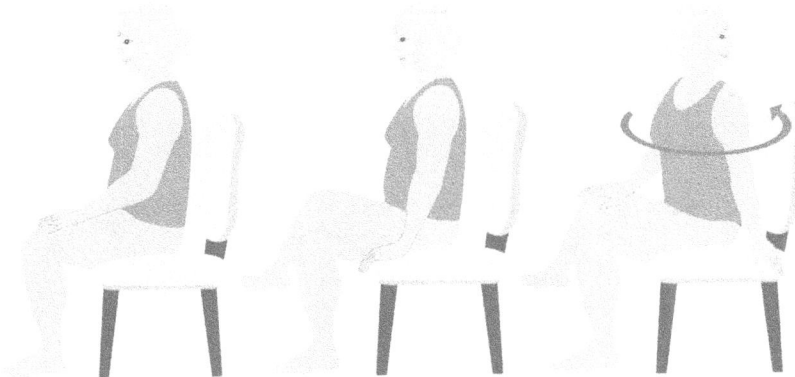

Steps:

1. Begin by sitting upright on a stable chair, with your feet flat on the floor.

2. Cross your left leg over your right, placing your left foot beside your right knee. This setup prepares your body for a deeper twist and stretch.

3. Place your right hand on your left knee and your left hand behind you on the chair. These hand placements aid in supporting the twist and ensuring stability.

4. Inhale deeply to prepare your body. As you exhale, gently twist your torso to the left, aiming to look over your left shoulder. This movement initiates the twist from your lower back, extending up through your spine to your neck.

5. Hold the position for a few breaths, allowing the twist to deepen gently with each exhale. Focus on feeling the stretch throughout your spine.

6. After holding, slowly return to the center before repeating the exercise on the opposite side. This ensures balanced flexibility and mobility in both directions.

Chair Cat-Cow Stretch

Helps with:	
» **Enhanced joint flexibility** The alternating movements of arching and rounding the back increase flexibility in the spine.	» **Improved posture** This exercise helps to correct and maintain proper spinal alignment.
» **Improved circulation** The flowing motion promotes blood flow throughout the spine and surrounding muscles.	» **Increased joint lubrication** The repetitive motion encourages the production of synovial fluid, enhancing joint lubrication.
Safety Precautions:	
-Move slowly and gently to avoid any strain. - If you have severe back pain or a spinal injury, consult with a healthcare provider before attempting this exercise.	

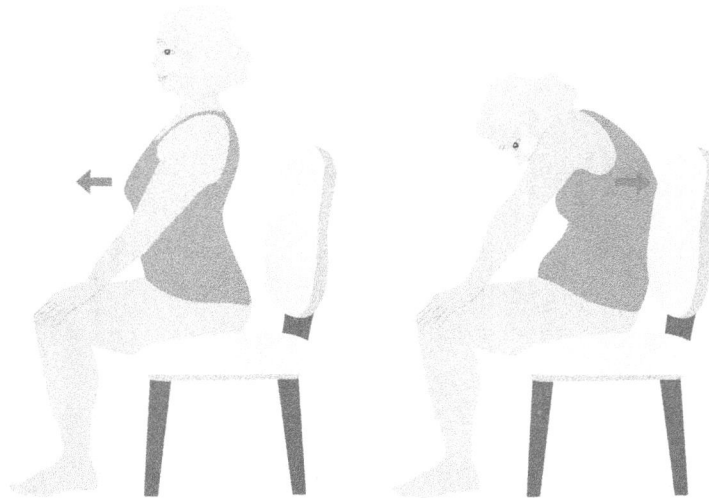

Steps:

1. Sit upright towards the front edge of a stable chair, placing your feet flat on the floor, hip-width apart. Place your hands on your knees or thighs for support.

2. Begin with the Cow pose: Inhale, arch your back, and tilt your pelvis back, sticking your buttocks out slightly. Lift your chest and chin upwards, gazing slightly forward or up, and pull your shoulders back. This position encourages a gentle arch in your lower back, opening the chest and stretching the front of your torso.

3. Transition to the Cat pose: Exhale, round your spine, and tilt your pelvis forward, tucking your tailbone under. Draw your chin towards your chest, gaze down at your navel,

and push your mid-back towards the chair back. This movement stretches the back of your spine and releases tension in your neck and shoulders.

4. Continue to flow smoothly between the Cow and Cat poses, following the rhythm of your breath: Inhale as you move into Cow pose, and exhale as you transition into Cat pose.

5. Repeat this sequence for several breath cycles (typically 5-10), focusing on the sensation of movement along your spine and the relaxation of tension with each transition.

Seated Forward Bend

Helps with:	
» **Enhanced joint flexibility** This pose stretches the spine, hips, and hamstrings, improving overall flexibility.	» **Pain reduction** It helps to relieve lower back pain by stretching and lengthening the spine.
» **Improved circulation** Forward bending increases blood flow to the spine and pelvic region.	» **Better muscle elasticity** Regular practice improves the elasticity of the muscles and connective tissues.
Safety Precautions:	
- Bend from your hips, not your waist. - Avoid if you have severe lower back issues.	

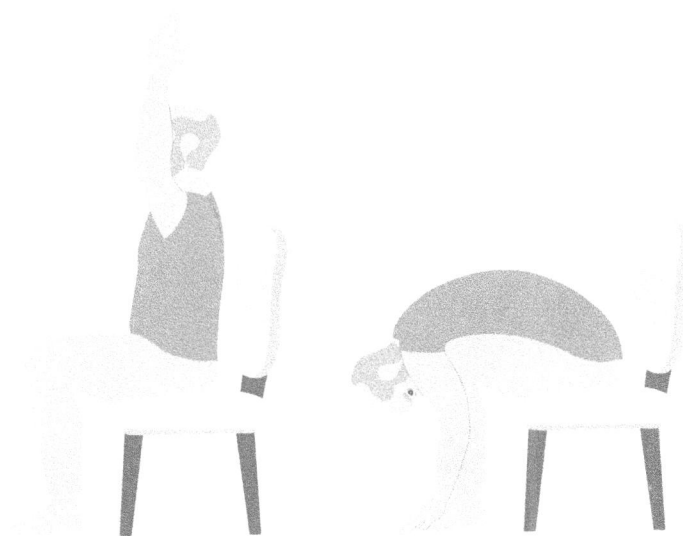

Steps:

1. Start by sitting upright on a secure chair. Keep your feet planted on the floor, ensuring they are parallel and hip-width apart for stability.

2. Inhale deeply and raise your arms overhead, bringing a gentle stretch to your upper body. This upward movement also aids in elongating the spine.

3. As you exhale, gradually hinge forward from your hips, not the waist. This distinction is crucial for targeting the right muscles and ensuring safety.

4. Extend your hands towards your feet or shins, depending on your comfort and flexibility. The key is to stretch without straining.

5. Hold this forward bend for a few deep breaths, allowing the stretch to penetrate your spine and lower back. Focus on the sensation of release in your back with each exhale.

6. To conclude, slowly rise back to the sitting position, using your hands for support if necessary.

Seated Shoulder Rolls

Helps with:	
» **Muscle strengthening** This exercise strengthens the muscles around the shoulders and upper back.	» **Improved circulation** The rolling motion promotes blood flow in the shoulder region.
» **Improved posture** It helps to correct rounded shoulders and improve overall posture.	» **Reduced muscle tension** Shoulder rolls help release tension and tightness in the shoulders and neck.
Safety Precautions:	
- Perform the movements slowly and gently to avoid any strain. - Keep your spine straight and aligned to prevent slouching during the exercise. - Breathe naturally, coordinating your breath with the movement for maximum relaxation.	

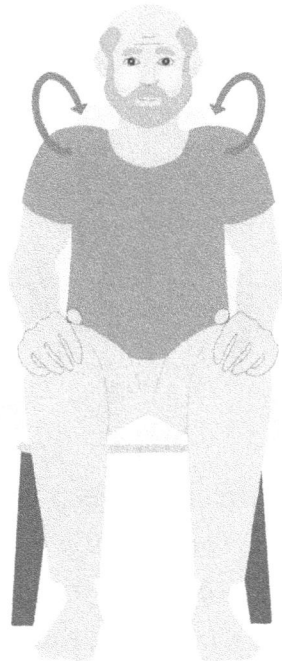

1. Begin by sitting upright in a chair with your feet flat on the floor, hip-width apart, ensuring a stable and grounded posture. Place your hands on your thighs or let them hang by your sides.

2. Inhale deeply, and as you exhale, slowly lift your shoulders towards your ears, initiating the rolling motion.

3. Continue the movement by gently rolling your shoulders back, drawing your shoulder blades towards each other to open up the chest.

4. As you complete the backward roll, start to lower your shoulders down, creating a circular motion.

5. Once your shoulders are in their lowest position, begin the next roll by lifting them towards your ears again, then forward, up, back, and down, reversing the direction of the rolls.

6. Perform this circular motion slowly and smoothly for several repetitions, typically 5-10 times in each direction, focusing on the sensation of release and relaxation in your shoulder and neck area.

7. Pause for a moment after completing the rolls in both directions, taking a few deep breaths to settle into the relaxation and openness created by the exercise.

Chair Lotus Pose Variation

Helps with:	
» **Enhanced joint flexibility** This pose gently stretches the hips, knees, and ankles, improving overall joint flexibility.	» **Muscle strengthening** Holding this pose strengthens the core and lower back muscles, providing stability and support.
» **Improved circulation** Sitting in this pose promotes blood flow to the lower body, enhancing overall circulation.	» **Better muscle elasticity** Regular practice improves the elasticity of the muscles and connective tissues around the hips and lower back.

Safety Precautions:
- Ensure movements into and out of the pose are gentle to avoid straining the hips, knees, or ankles.
- Listen to your body and adjust the pose as necessary to avoid discomfort.

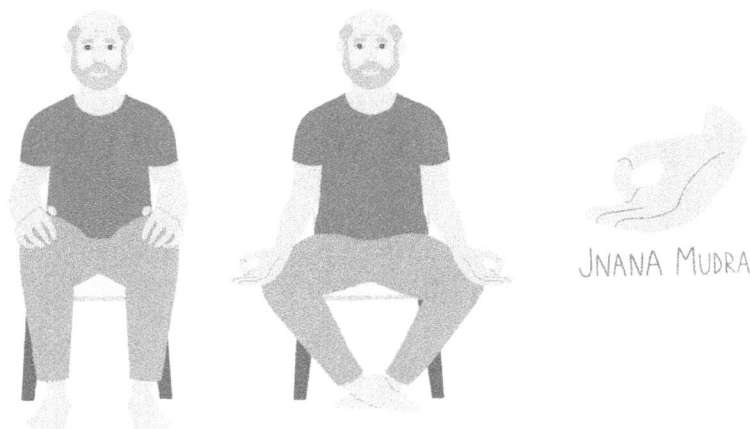

JNANA MUDRA

<u>Steps:</u>

1. Start seated comfortably towards the front of a stable chair, keeping your feet flat on the floor to start. Ensure your spine is erect, promoting an aligned posture.

2. Gently cross your ankles in front of you, allowing them to stay close to the floor. This position should create a mild, comfortable stretch in the hips without the intensity of the full Lotus position.

3. Bring the backs of your hands to rest on your knees. Form Jnana Mudra by touching each thumb to its respective index finger, creating a circle, while keeping the rest of your fingers extended. This mudra is known for promoting wisdom and concentration.

4. With your ankles crossed and hands in Jnana Mudra, sit tall and breathe deeply. Allow your shoulders to relax away from your ears, and close your eyes if comfortable to enhance the meditative aspect of the pose.

5. Stay in this pose for several deep breaths, focusing on the sensation of relaxation and openness in your hips and lower back. Use this time to cultivate a sense of inner peace and calm.

6. To release, gently uncross your ankles and place your feet flat on the floor. Relax your hands and take a moment to notice any sensations in your body.

Chair Wrist Stretch

<u>Helps with:</u>	
» **Enhanced joint flexibility** This pose strengthens and stretches the legs and hips, reducing joint pain and improving stability.	» **Pain reduction** It encourages good spinal alignment and strengthens the core muscles, supporting spinal health.

» **Improved circulation**	» **Increased joint lubrication**
Stretching the wrists promotes blood flow to the hands and fingers.	Stretching encourages the production of synovial fluid, enhancing joint lubrication.

Safety Precautions:

- Perform the stretch gently to avoid overextension or strain on the wrists.
- If you experience any pain or discomfort during the stretch, ease up on the intensity or discontinue the stretch.
- Keep your movements slow and controlled, especially when extending your arms and pressing your palms forward.

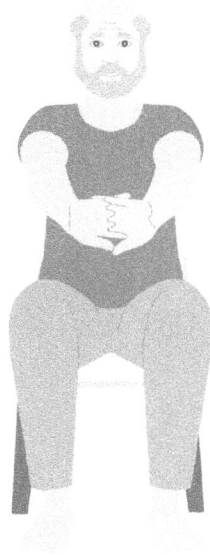

Steps:

1. Begin in a comfortable seated ensuring your spine is straight and shoulders are relaxed.
2. Gently interlace your fingers in front of you, ensuring a comfortable grip without squeezing too tightly.
3. With your fingers interlaced, flip your palms to face forward, away from your body. This action begins the process of engaging the wrists and forearms.
4. Carefully lift your arms to shoulder height, maintaining the interlaced fingers and forward-facing palms. Ensure your shoulders remain relaxed and down, away from your ears.
5. As you straighten your arms, press your palms forward, feeling a gentle stretch in the wrists and forearms. Ensure your arms are parallel to the floor, and you're pressing out as if against an invisible barrier.
6. Maintain this position for 5 deep breaths, focusing on the sensation of stretching and opening in the wrists and forearms. With each exhale, try to deepen the stretch slightly, without causing discomfort.

7. After holding for 5 breaths, gently release the interlace of your fingers and lower your arms back to your sides or lap. Shake out your hands and wrists gently if it feels comfortable.

Seated Pigeon Pose

Helps with:	
» **Enhanced joint flexibility** This pose deeply stretches the hips and glutes, improving flexibility.	» **Pain reduction** It helps to alleviate pain in the hips and lower back by releasing tension in the gluteal muscles.
» **Improved balance and coordination** Stretching and opening the hips enhances overall balance and stability.	» **Better muscle elasticity** Regular practice improves the elasticity of the muscles around the hips and lower back.

Safety Precautions:

- Be gentle to avoid stress on the knee.
- Avoid if you have severe hip or knee issues.

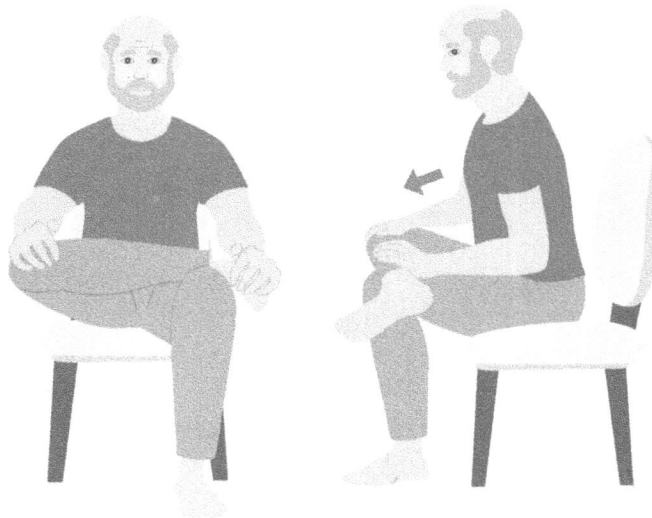

Steps:

1. Start by sitting upright in a chair, ensuring your feet are grounded on the floor for a stable base.

2. Gently place your right ankle on your left thigh, just above the knee, creating a figure-four shape. This position initiates the stretch in the hips and glutes.

3. Allow your right knee to relax, avoiding any forceful pressing. For a deeper stretch, gently apply pressure to your right knee with your hand, increasing the stretch in the outer hip and thigh.

4. Slowly lean forward, bending at the hips while keeping your spine straight and tall until you feel a stretch in your lower back.

5. Hold this position for several breaths, focusing on deep, steady breathing to facilitate relaxation and deepen the stretch.

6. Carefully release your leg and switch to the other side, repeating the pose to ensure balanced flexibility and relief in both hips.

Sticking with it is key, my friends. When you make these carefully chosen chair yoga exercises a regular part of your routine, you're doing more than just stretching and moving—you're investing in your future comfort and mobility. Little by little, you'll feel those stiff joints loosening up and those tight muscles starting to relax. You'll notice everyday activities becoming easier, and soon enough, you'll be moving through your day with more ease and confidence.

These exercises don't just address specific areas of stiffness; they enhance your overall well-being. Better joint health and increased flexibility can transform your life, leading to more activity, independence, and fulfillment. So, keep at it. Every bit of progress you make brings you closer to greater physical freedom and a higher quality of life. Let's turn those everyday movements into effortless actions and keep you moving smoothly and confidently.

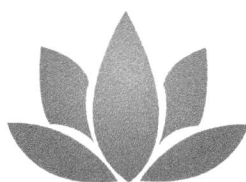

CHAPTER 5
CHAIR YOGA FOR MUSCLE STRENGTHENING AND ELASTICITY

Alright, let's talk about strength. As we age, maintaining muscle strength is crucial for supporting our joints and ensuring overall mobility. Strong muscles are the foundation of our bodies, providing the stability we need to move confidently and reducing the risk of falls and injuries. This chapter is all about exercises that build and maintain vital muscle strength, helping you improve daily functioning and perform everyday tasks with ease.

The exercises in this chapter are specifically designed to be accessible and effective for seniors. They promote gradual progress and sustained strength, ensuring that you can safely and effectively enhance your muscle elasticity. With stronger, more elastic muscles, your body becomes more resilient and adaptable, making it easier to handle the physical demands of daily life. But it's not just about the physical benefits—building muscle strength also boosts your confidence and independence, empowering you to lead a more active and fulfilling life.

Chair Assisted Leg Lifts

Helps with:	
» **Muscle strengthening** Builds strength in the lower body, focusing on the quadriceps, hip flexors & core.	» **Improved balance and coordination** Strengthening the legs and core enhances overall stability and coordination.

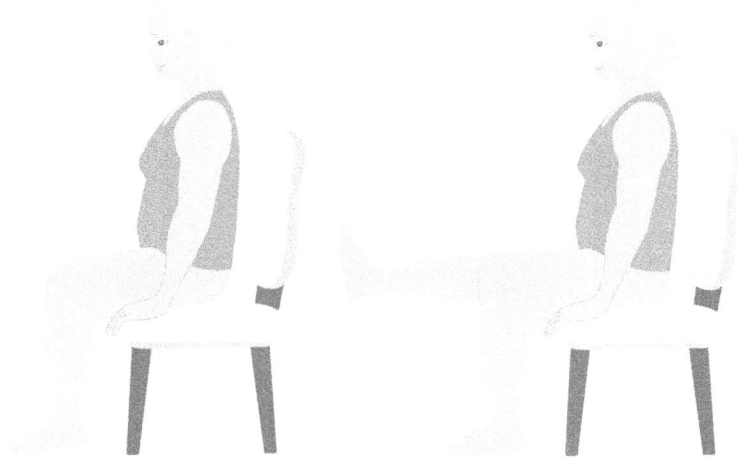

Steps:

1. Begin by sitting upright in a stable chair, ensuring your feet are flat on the ground. This starting position promotes good posture and prepares your body for the exercise.

2. Grasp the sides of the chair lightly for support. This not only aids in maintaining balance during the exercise but also ensures safety and control.

3. Carefully extend one leg out in front of you, striving to keep it parallel to the floor. The goal is to activate the muscles in your thigh and core without straining them.

4. Hold this extended position for a few seconds, focusing on engaging the thigh muscles while keeping the rest of your body stable.

5. Gently lower the leg back to the starting position, controlling the movement to maximize the exercise's benefits.

6. Perform 5-10 repetitions with each leg, alternating to ensure balanced strength and flexibility in both legs.

Seated Calf Raises

Helps with:	
» **Muscle strengthening** This exercise strengthens the calf muscles, improving lower leg strength.	» **Improved balance and coordination** Strengthening the calves enhances stability and coordination in the lower body.

» **Improved circulation** The up-and-down motion promotes blood flow to the lower legs and feet.	

Safety Precautions:
- Move slowly and avoid jerky movements. - If you have ankle or calf injuries, proceed with caution.

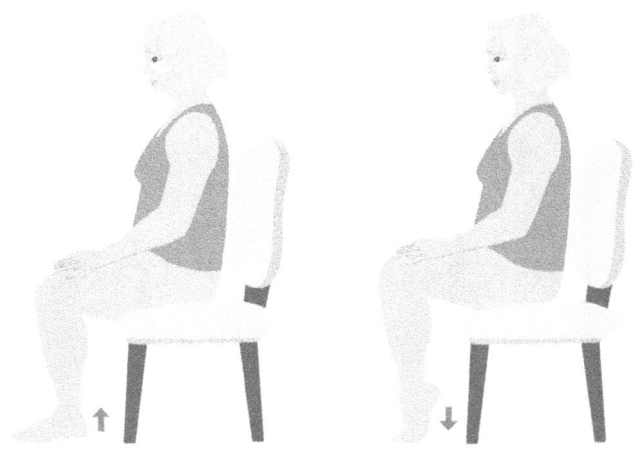

Steps:

1. Start by sitting upright in a chair with your feet flat on the floor. Ensure your posture is straight, supporting overall alignment and balance.

2. Gradually raise your heels off the floor, shifting your weight onto the balls of your feet. This movement engages the calf muscles, promoting strength and stability.

3. Hold this raised position for a few seconds. This pause is key to maximizing muscle engagement and enhancing stability in the ankles.

4. Gently lower your heels back to the floor, controlling the movement to ensure smooth and steady strengthening.

5. Repeat the calf raise 10-15 times. This repetition range is optimal for building strength and endurance in the calf muscles and ankles.

Seated Leg Stretches

Helps with:	
» **Enhanced joint flexibility** Seated leg stretches improve flexibility in the hamstrings, calves, and hips, making it easier to perform daily activities with greater ease and comfort.	» **Muscle strengthening** These stretches engage and strengthen the muscles of the legs, particularly the quadriceps and hamstrings, providing better support for the knees and hips.

» **Improved circulation**	» **Better muscle elasticity**
Stretching the legs promotes better blood flow, enhancing circulation throughout the lower body and reducing the risk of blood clots.	Consistent stretching improves the elasticity of the leg muscles and connective tissues, making them more pliable and resilient.

Safety Precautions:

- Do not overstretch; go only as far as comfortable.
- Avoid if you have severe sciatica.

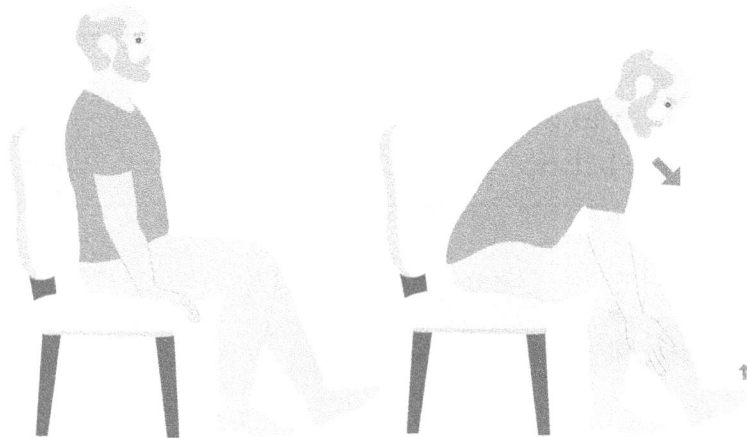

Steps:

1. Start by sitting on the edge of a stable chair, ensuring your posture is upright. This initial position helps maintain balance and alignment for an effective stretch.

2. Fully extend one leg forward, resting the heel on the ground and toes pointing upwards. If you find it challenging, it's perfectly fine to keep a slight bend in the knee. This position targets the hamstring and calf of the extended leg.

3. Keep the other foot flat on the floor to support balance and stability.

4. Inhale deeply to prepare. As you exhale, gently lean forward from your hips towards the extended leg. This forward motion enhances the stretch in the hamstring and lower back. Move into the stretch only as far as comfortable, avoiding any strain.

5. Hold the position for a few breaths, allowing the stretch to deepen gently with each exhale. This not only aids in flexibility but also promotes relaxation.

6. After holding, gently return to the starting position and switch legs, repeating the stretch to ensure balanced flexibility on both sides.

Chair Warrior Variation III

Helps with:	
» **Muscle strengthening** This pose strengthens the legs, core, and lower back, enhancing overall lower body and core strength.	» **Improved balance and coordination** Balancing on one leg while extending the other behind improves stability and coordination.
» **Enhanced joint flexibility** Stretching the legs and engaging the core improves flexibility in the hips and lower back.	» **Better muscle elasticity** Consistent practice of this pose improves the elasticity of the leg and core muscles, making them more pliable and resilient.

Safety Precautions:

- Use the chair for support to maintain balance.
- Avoid if you have severe balance issues.

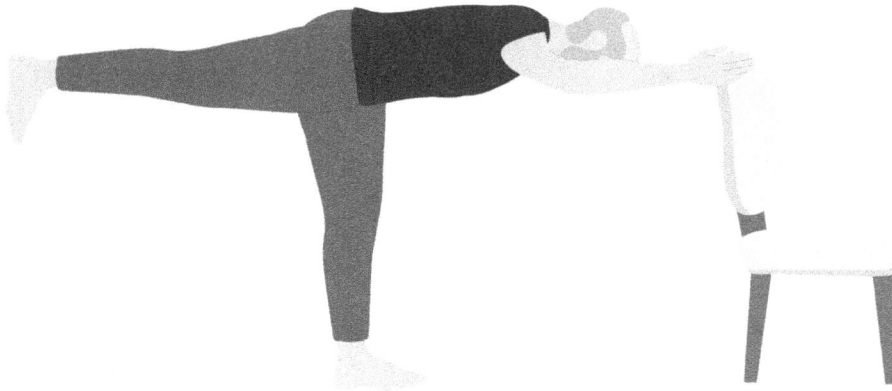

Steps:

1. Begin by standing behind a chair, placing your hands securely on the backrest. This provides the necessary support to perform the pose safely, especially for those concerned with balance.

2. Carefully lift your right leg straight behind you. At the same time, lean your torso forward until your body forms a 'T' shape. This action engages the muscles in your standing leg and core, challenging your balance and strengthening these areas.

3. Extend your arms forward, keeping them parallel to the floor. This arm position helps with balance and aligns your body correctly in the pose.

4. Hold this position for several deep breaths, focusing on maintaining stability and alignment. The act of balancing and focusing during this pose enhances concentration and mental clarity.

5. Gently return to your starting position and repeat the exercise with your left leg lifted. This ensures that both sides of the body are worked evenly, maintaining symmetry in muscle strength and flexibility.

Seated Knee Extensions

Helps with:	
» **Muscle strengthening** This exercise targets the quadriceps, building strength in the thigh muscles.	» **Improved joint flexibility** Extending and bending the knee enhances flexibility in the knee joint.
» **Pain reduction** Strengthening the muscles around the knee can help reduce pain and improve joint stability.	
Safety Precautions:	
- Extend your knee gently. - Avoid if you have severe knee pain.	

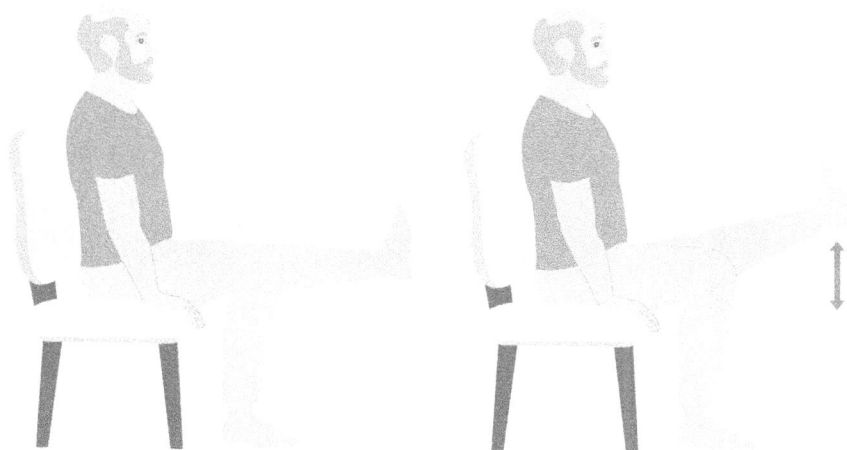

Steps:

1. Begin by sitting upright on a chair, ensuring your feet are firmly on the ground.
2. Extend one leg out in front of you, preparing for the lift. This action sets the stage for strengthening the muscles around your knee.
3. Slowly raise and lower the extended leg, maintaining a smooth and controlled movement. This precision helps in maximizing muscle engagement while protecting the knee joint.
4. Aim for 10-15 lifts, focusing on the quality of movement rather than speed. Each lift contributes to building strength in the thigh muscles and improving flexibility in the knee joint.

5. After completing the set, switch to the other leg to ensure balanced strengthening across both legs.

Supported Chair Pose

Helps with:	
» **Muscle strengthening** This pose strengthens the legs, glutes, and core, building overall lower body strength.	» **Improved balance and coordination** Engaging the core and maintaining balance in the pose enhances stability.
» **Improved posture** The pose encourages proper spinal alignment and strengthens postural muscles.	
Safety Precautions:	
-Keep your back straight and avoid leaning too far forward. - Avoid if you have knee problems.	

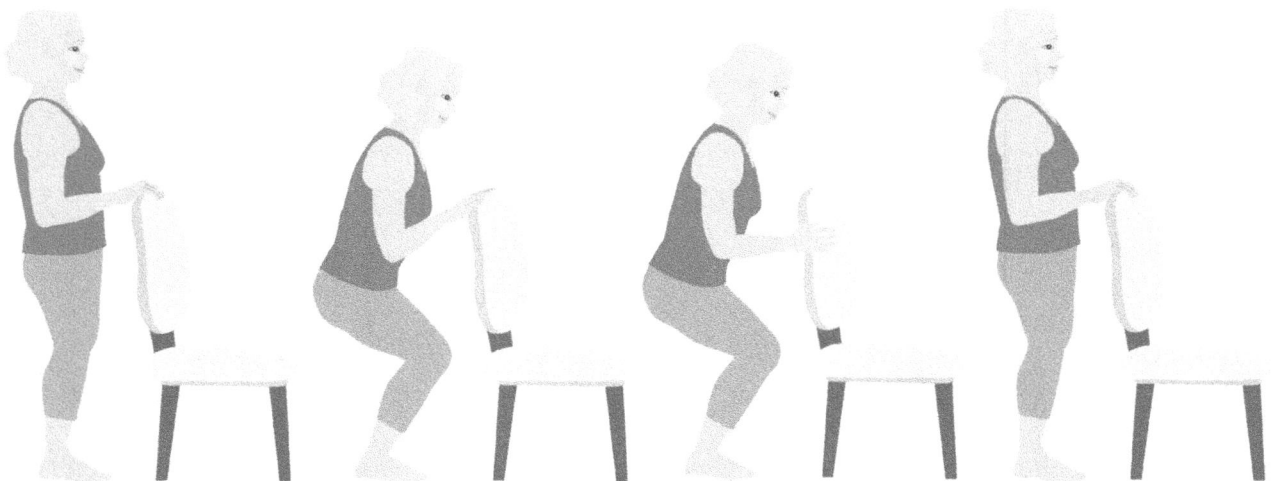

Steps:

1. Begin by standing in front of the back of your chair, placing your hands lightly on the top for initial support. Ensure your feet are shoulder-width apart and firmly on the ground for stability.

2. Take a deep breath in, engaging your core to keep your spine long and protected as you start to bend your knees. Imagine you're about to sit down, initiating a controlled descent.

3. As you lower your body, shift your grip to the sides of the chair backrest for added stability. Lower yourself to a comfortable depth, ideally until your thighs are about parallel to the floor, creating a stable base without straining.

4. Ensure your knees remain aligned with your toes, avoiding any inward or outward drifting. This alignment helps protect your joints. Maintain this squat position for five breaths, focusing on stability and the engagement of your leg muscles.

5. To rise, press down through your feet, using the strength of your legs and core to return to a standing position.

Seated Sun Salutation Flow II

Helps with:	
» **Muscle strengthening** This sequence engages various muscle groups, building strength in the arms, legs, and core.	» **Improved circulation** The dynamic movements promote blood flow throughout the body.
» **Improved balance and coordination** Coordinating breath with movement enhances overall stability and coordination.	» **Reduced muscle tension** The flowing sequence helps to release tension in the muscles.
Safety Precautions: -Move through the sequence at a pace that feels comfortable, avoiding any movements that cause discomfort. - Keep movements smooth and controlled to prevent strain.	

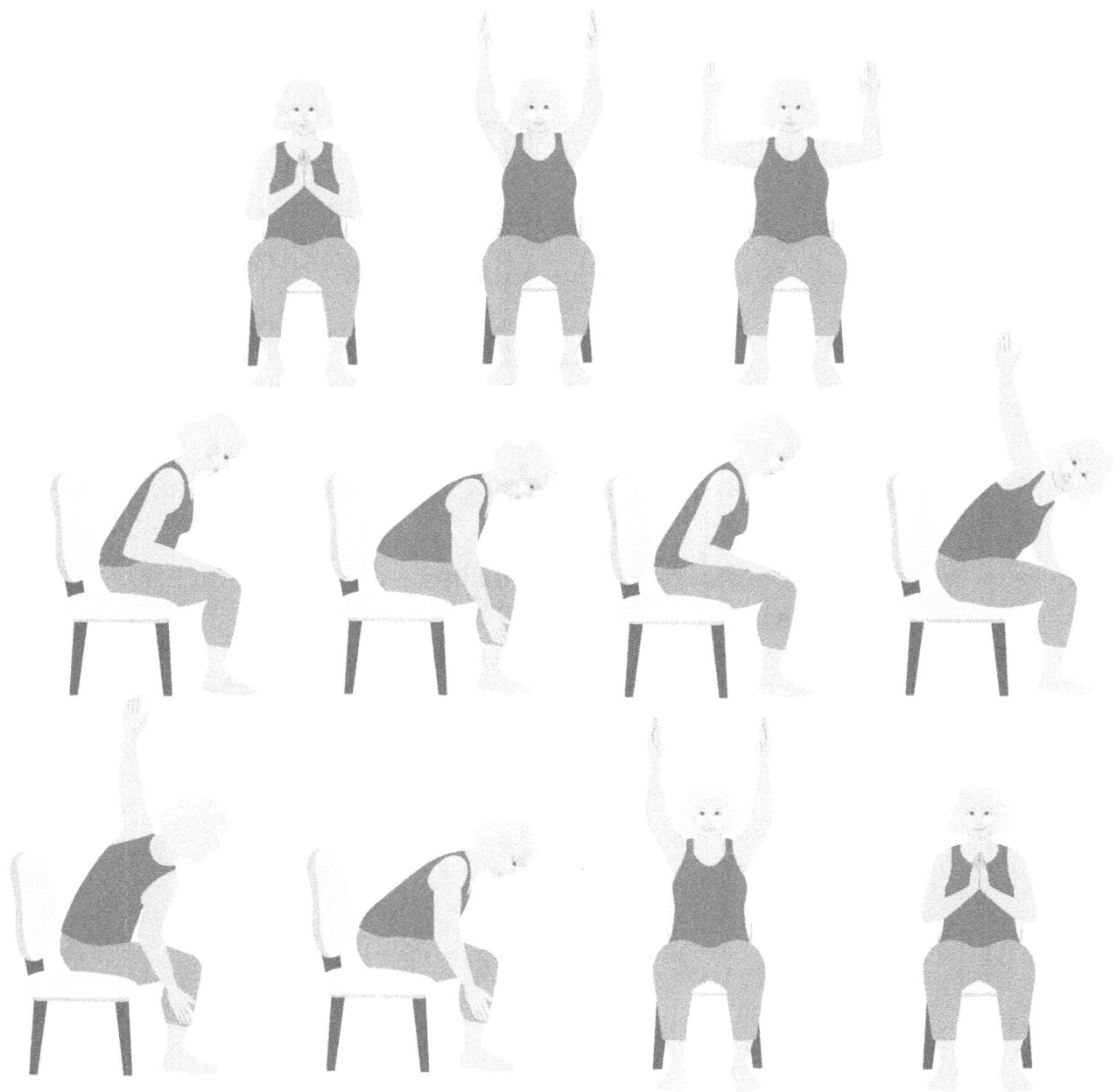

Steps:

1. Begin by sitting upright on your chair. Bring your hands to your heart, sitting tall and establishing a sense of grounding.

2. Open your arms to the sides and then move them all the way up overhead. As you reach the top, turn your hands so that your palms are facing forward.

3. Lower your arms to shoulder height, adopting the Cactus arms pose.

4. Lean forward halfway from your hips, pause, and then bring your hands to rest on your kneecaps. You have the option to keep your hands here or slowly slide them down your legs as you fold forward. Extend as far as feels comfortable, honoring your body's limits.

5. Lift halfway up, bringing your hands back to your knees for support.

6. Fold forward once more, and as you inhale, extend your right hand up, turning your head to look towards your right hand, while keeping your left hand on your left leg.

7. Exhale and lower your right hand, then inhale and switch, extending your left hand up to stretch the other side, turning your head to follow the movement.

8. Exhale, bring your left hand down, and as you inhale, lift your head and extend your arms to the side, reaching up, then bring your hands down to your heart.

9. Repeat this flow 3-5 times, moving with your breath and focusing on the fluidity and ease of the sequence.

Consistency is your best friend here. By regularly practicing these targeted chair yoga exercises, you're not just building muscle—you're investing in your long-term mobility and independence. Over time, you'll notice your muscles becoming stronger and more elastic, which will support your joints and improve your overall stability. This means more confidence in your movements and a greater ability to enjoy your daily activities without fear of injury.

These exercises will contribute to your overall mobility, stability, and resilience. With each session, you're empowering yourself to lead a more active, independent, and fulfilling life. Remember, every bit of progress counts. Let's work together to strengthen those muscles, improve your elasticity, and support your joint health. Keep at it, and you'll be amazed at the difference it makes in your everyday life. You've got this!

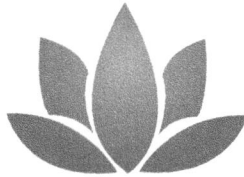

CHAPTER 6
CHAIR YOGA FOR PAIN REDUCTION AND TENSION RELIEF

Let's face it, pain can be a real obstacle to enjoying life, especially when it affects the upper body and shoulders. Whether it's from cervical spondylosis, a herniated disc, muscle strain, rotator cuff injuries, frozen shoulder, or bursitis, dealing with pain can feel overwhelming. But here's the good news: chair yoga offers gentle yet effective exercises specifically designed to relieve these types of pain and tension.

This chapter is all about targeting those troublesome areas and providing relief. We'll focus on gentle movements that help alleviate pain in the spine, neck, shoulders, and upper body. These exercises are accessible to everyone, ensuring you can perform them safely and effectively. By incorporating these stretches and movements into your routine, you can reduce pain and tension, making your day-to-day activities more comfortable and enjoyable.

Chair Revolved Triangle Pose

Helps with:	
» **Reduced muscle tension** This pose targets the muscles in the lower back, hips, and legs, helping to release tightness and tension. The twisting motion helps to unwind tight muscles along the spine, providing a deep stretch that reduces overall muscle tension.	» **Pain reduction** This pose stretches and lengthens the spine, hips, and hamstrings, helping to alleviate pain in the lower back, hips, and legs. By gently twisting the spine, this pose helps to relieve tension and pressure on the spinal discs, which can reduce pain in the back and neck.
» **Improved circulation** Twisting and stretching the body in this pose promotes better blood flow to the spine, hips, and legs, enhancing overall circulation. Improved circulation can help reduce inflammation and speed up the healing process, further alleviating pain and tension.	» **Improved posture** It encourages proper spinal alignment and strengthens the muscles that support good posture. By promoting better posture, this pose can help prevent and reduce pain associated with poor alignment and muscle imbalances.

Safety Precautions:

- Move into the twist slowly to avoid strain.
- Use the chair for support to maintain balance.

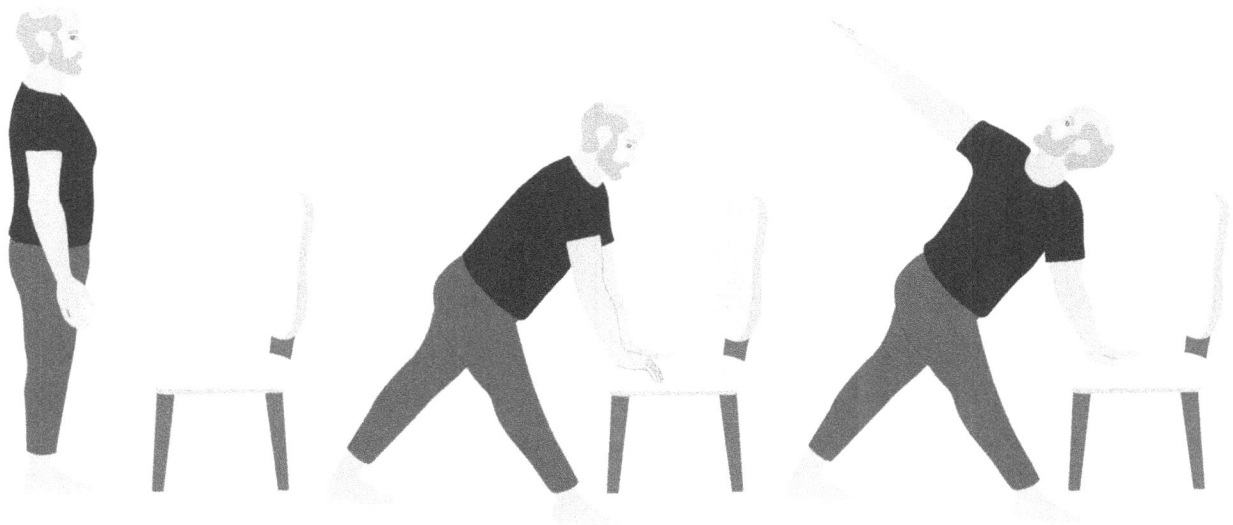

1. Begin by standing in front of a chair, feet hip-width apart, facing towards the chair.

2. Step your left foot back about a leg's length, keeping your right foot facing forward. The back foot should be at a 45-degree angle, grounding through the edge of the foot.

3. Inhale and extend your torso over the right leg, placing your hands on the seat of the chair for support. This initial forward bend helps to lengthen the spine and prepare for the twist.

4. As you exhale, initiate the twist to your right, extending your right arm towards the ceiling if balance allows. Your left hand can remain on the chair for support, or for a deeper twist, place it on the outside of your right foot on the chair.

5. Turn your head to gaze up towards your right hand, ensuring your spine is elongated and your twist originates from your mid-torso.

6. Hold the pose for several breaths, focusing on deepening the twist with each exhale while maintaining balance and stability.

7. To come out of the pose, lower your right arm, unwind your torso, and gently stand back up to the starting position.

8. Repeat on the opposite side to maintain balance in the body.

Chair Downward Dog Pose

Helps with:	
» **Pain reduction** It stretches the entire back, including the spine, shoulders, and hamstrings, helping to alleviate pain and discomfort in these areas. By lengthening the spine and reducing compression, it can relieve pressure on the lower back.	» **Reduced muscle tension** This pose helps release tightness and tension in the back, shoulders, and legs. The stretch targets large muscle groups, providing a deep release and relaxation, which can reduce overall muscle tension.
» **Improved circulation** The inverted position of this pose encourages blood flow to the upper body, promoting better circulation. Improved circulation helps deliver oxygen and nutrients to muscles and joints, aiding in recovery and reducing inflammation.	» **Improved posture** Engaging the core and aligning the spine in this pose promotes proper posture. Strengthening the muscles that support good posture helps prevent slouching and reduces the risk of developing pain associated with poor alignment.
Safety Precautions:	
- Ensure the chair is stable. - Avoid if you have severe wrist or shoulder pain.	

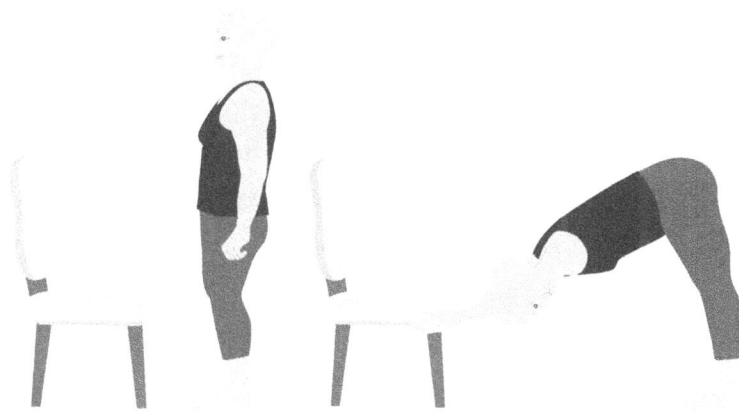

<u>Steps:</u>

1. Begin by standing in front of a chair, feet hip-width apart, ensuring the chair is stable and secure. This precaution is crucial for maintaining safety throughout the pose.

2. Lean forward and place your hands on the seat of the chair. Carefully step back until your body forms an inverted 'V' shape. This positioning uses the chair to support your upper body, making the pose accessible and safe.

3. Aim to keep your spine and legs straight, creating a long line from your hands through your spine and down to your hips. This alignment helps in stretching the back and legs effectively.

4. Gently press your chest towards your thighs, deepening the stretch along your back and hamstrings. This movement also aids in strengthening your arms by bearing some of your body's weight.

5. Hold this position for several deep breaths, focusing on the stretch and the calming rhythm of your breathing. The duration of the hold helps in maximizing the stretch and the calming benefits of the pose.

6. To release, slowly walk your feet forward, coming back to a standing position and then relax. This gradual movement helps in avoiding any sudden strain on the muscles.

Seated Extended Side Angle Pose

<u>Helps with:</u>	
» **Pain reduction** This pose stretches the sides of the body, including the hips, waist, and lower back. By elongating these muscles, it helps to relieve tension and alleviate pain, particularly in the lower back and hips.	» **Reduced muscle tension** The stretch targets the obliques, hip flexors, and lower back, helping to release tightness and reduce overall muscle tension. Regular practice can help keep these muscles relaxed and less prone to stiffness.

» **Enhanced joint flexibility**	» **Improved posture**
This pose increases flexibility in the hips, spine, and shoulders. Enhanced flexibility can improve overall mobility and reduce the risk of injury.	By engaging the core and aligning the spine during the stretch, this pose helps promote proper posture. Strengthening the muscles that support good posture helps prevent slouching and reduces the risk of developing pain associated with poor alignment.

Safety Precautions:

- Ensure the chair is stable and secure to prevent it from moving during the pose.
- Move into and out of the pose gently to avoid any sudden movements that could lead to discomfort or injury.
- Listen to your body and only stretch as far as comfortably possible without straining.

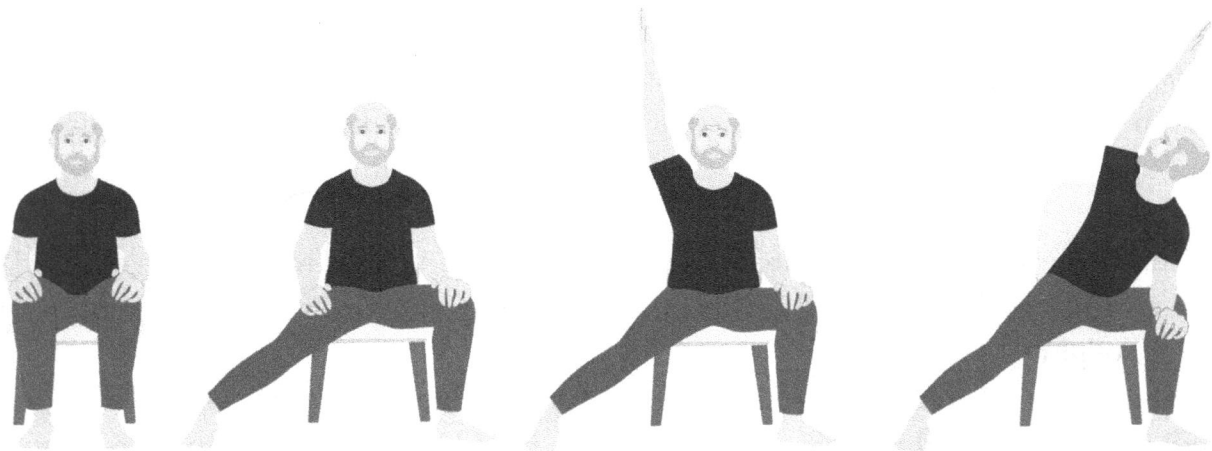

Steps:

1. Begin by sitting upright in a chair, feet flat on the floor, spaced hip-width apart. Ensure your back is straight, and you're positioned towards the front of the chair for greater freedom of movement.

2. Extend your right leg out to the side, keeping your left foot planted firmly on the ground opening your hips as far as it feels comfortable. If possible, rotate your right foot so that it points slightly outward, aligning with the direction of your stretch.

3. Inhale and raise your right arm overhead, extending it alongside your ear. Keep your left hand on your left thigh.

4. As you exhale, gently lean your torso to the left, gently resting your forearm over the left thigh. Extend your right arm further to enhance the stretch along the right side of your

body. Keep your chest open and your gaze directed forward or slightly upwards, maintaining a long, straight line from your right fingertips down to your right hip.

5. Maintain this position for several deep breaths, focusing on the stretch along the right side of your torso. With each exhale, try to deepen the stretch slightly, without pushing beyond your comfort level.

6. To release, inhale and gently come back to an upright seated position, lowering your right arm. Bring your right leg back to the starting position.

7. Repeat on the Opposite Side: Extend your left leg out, and repeat the stretch on the other side to ensure balance in the stretch and flexibility.

Seated Wide Leg Forward

Helps with:	
» **Pain reduction** This pose stretches the inner thighs, hamstrings, and lower back, which can help alleviate pain and discomfort in these areas. By lengthening and releasing tension in the muscles, it reduces strain on the lower back and hips, providing relief from chronic pain.	» **Reduced muscle tension** The deep stretch provided by this pose helps release tightness and tension in the inner thighs, hamstrings, and lower back. Regular practice can help keep these muscles relaxed and reduce the overall feeling of stiffness.
» **Improved circulation** Stretching the legs and lower back promotes better blood flow to these areas. Improved circulation helps deliver oxygen and nutrients to muscles and joints, aiding in recovery and reducing inflammation.	» **Improved posture** By engaging the core and aligning the spine during the stretch, this pose helps promote proper posture. Strengthening the muscles that support good posture helps prevent slouching and reduces the risk of developing pain associated with poor alignment.
Safety Precautions:	
- Move into the forward bend slowly to avoid straining the back. - If you have hip or hamstring issues, moderate the stretch.	

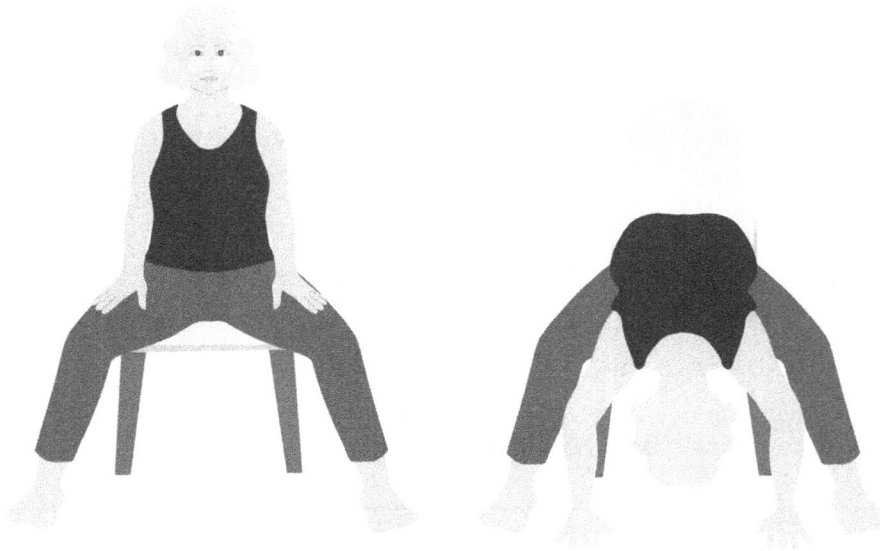

Steps:

1. Begin by sitting on the edge of your chair, providing the freedom to open your legs wide without restriction. This starting position is essential for achieving the maximum benefit from the stretch.

2. Take a deep breath in to prepare, focusing on elongating your spine. As you exhale, gently hinge forward from your hips, leading with your chest. This technique ensures a safe and effective stretch that targets the intended areas without straining the back.

3. Lower your torso towards the floor as far as it feels comfortable for you, allowing your hands to rest either on the floor or on your legs. This variation allows for personalization of the stretch based on your current flexibility and comfort level.

4. Maintain this forward bend for several deep breaths, embracing the stretch and the calming effect it has on your mind. The duration of the hold is a crucial aspect, providing ample time for the muscles to relax and lengthen.

5. To conclude the pose, slowly rise back up to a seated position, taking care to move gently to prevent any sudden strain on the back or legs.

Seated Catcus Arms

Helps with:	
» **Pain reduction** This pose opens up the chest and shoulders, helping to alleviate pain and discomfort in these areas.	» **Reduced muscle tension** Stretching the chest and shoulder muscles helps release tightness and reduce muscle tension.

| » **Improved posture** | |
| This pose encourages proper alignment of the spine and shoulders, promoting better overall posture. | |
| <td colspan="2">Safety Precautions:</td> |
| <td colspan="2">- Move within a comfortable range to avoid shoulder discomfort.
- Keep your spine neutral to prevent undue strain on the back.</td> |

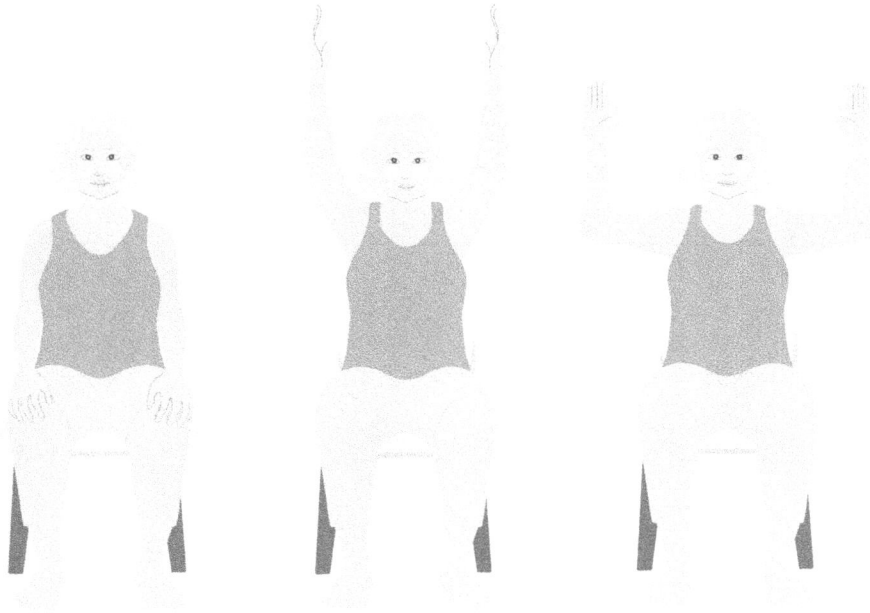

Steps:

1. Sit upright on a chair with feet flat on the ground, shoulder-width apart, providing a stable and supportive base.

2. Raise both arms towards the ceiling while engaging your core to stabilize your shoulders and ribcage.

3. Gently tuck your chin to maintain alignment of your head with your spine, avoiding forward head posture.

4. Exhale and bend your elbows, lowering your arms until they are parallel to the floor, with palms facing forward. Draw your shoulder blades together and gently lift your chest, creating the cactus arm shape.

5. Inhale and extend your arms back towards the ceiling, keeping your core engaged for stability and support.

6. Perform this bending and straightening motion 3-5 times, focusing on the movement's smoothness and the sensation of stretching and strengthening.

Chair Mountain Pose with Chest Opener

Helps with:	
» **Pain reduction** This pose opens up the chest and stretches the front of the shoulders, relieving tightness and discomfort. » **Improved posture** Opening the chest encourages proper spinal alignment and improves overall posture.	» **Reduced muscle tension** Stretching the chest and shoulder muscles helps release tightness and reduce muscle tension.
Safety Precautions:	
- Keep your back straight and avoid overextending. - If you have balance issues, ensure the chair is stable.	

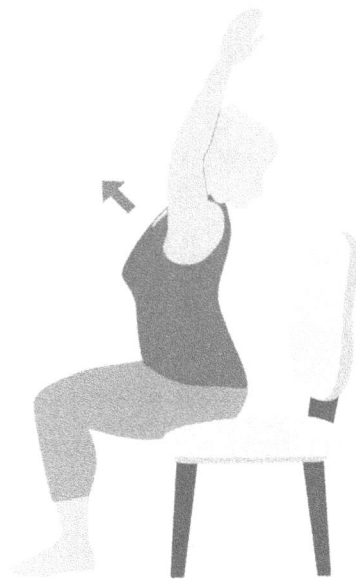

Steps:

1. Begin by sitting at the edge of your chair, ensuring your feet are planted firmly on the ground and your arms rest comfortably at your sides.

2. With an inhalation, lift your arms above your head, allowing your palms to face each other, reaching towards the sky.

3. As you exhale, allow your back to gently arch, opening up your chest to the world and slightly tilting your head back, as if basking in the glow of the sun.

4. Engage the muscles in your thighs, feeling a connection through your legs, and elongate your spine as if a string is pulling you upwards.

5. Maintain this pose for a few deep breaths, feeling the stretch and openness in your body.
6. On an exhale, slowly lower your arms back to your sides, returning to your starting position with a sense of renewal and strength.

Seated Arm Circles

Helps with:	
» **Pain reduction** This exercise loosens up the shoulders and arms, helping to relieve pain and discomfort in these areas. » **Improved circulation** Arm circles promote blood flow to the shoulders and arms, enhancing overall circulation.	» **Reduced muscle tension** The circular motion helps release tightness in the shoulder and arm muscles.
Safety Precautions:	
- Keep your movements slow and controlled to avoid any strain on your shoulders. - If you experience any pain or discomfort, reduce the size of your circles or take a break.	

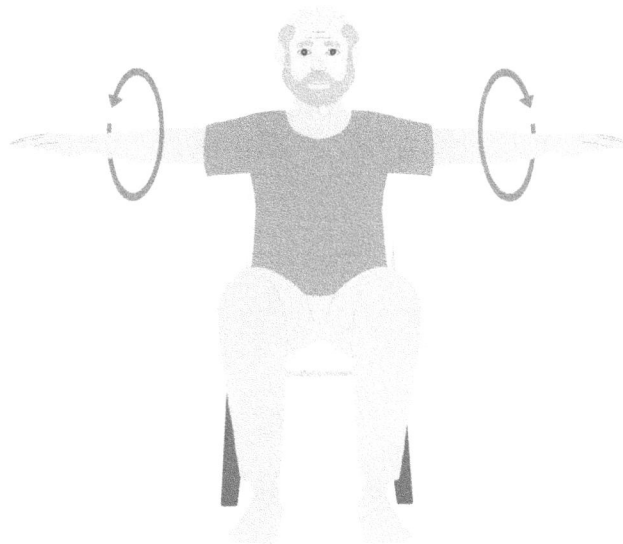

Steps:

1. Begin by sitting upright in a chair, with your feet flat on the ground.
2. Extend your arms out to the sides at shoulder height, keeping them straight. Ensure your palms are facing down to start, positioning your body in a T-shape.

3. Start making small circles with your arms, moving them in a forward motion. Focus on keeping the circles controlled and your arms level with your shoulders.

4. Gradually increase the size of the circles as you become more comfortable, ensuring you maintain control and do not strain your shoulder muscles.

5. After 15 seconds or when you're ready, reverse the direction of your circles, moving your arms in a backward motion. This change in direction helps to engage different muscles in your shoulders and upper back.

6. Continue performing the arm circles for a total of 30 seconds to 1 minute, alternating between forward and backward motions. You can adjust the duration based on your comfort and fitness level.

7. As you perform the arm circles, remember to breathe deeply and evenly. Proper breathing enhances oxygen flow to your muscles and helps keep you relaxed and focused.

Pain and tension don't have to control your life. By regularly practicing these chair yoga exercises, you can find relief and improve your overall quality of life. These gentle movements are designed to target the specific areas where pain and tension often reside, helping you to loosen up and feel more at ease.

Consistency is key. Make these exercises a part of your daily routine and watch as the pain starts to diminish and your mobility improves. You'll not only feel better physically but also gain a sense of empowerment and control over your well-being. Let's work together to reduce pain, relieve tension, and keep you moving comfortably and confidently.

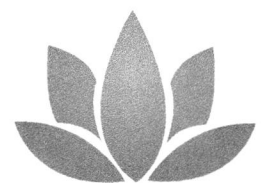

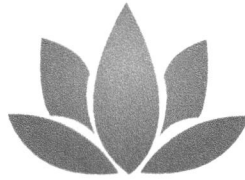

CHAPTER 7
CHAIR YOGA FOR STABILITY AND BALANCE

As we age, maintaining stability and balance becomes crucial for preventing falls and ensuring overall mobility. Falls can lead to serious injuries that significantly impact a senior's quality of life and independence. That's why this chapter is dedicated to exercises designed to improve your stability and balance. These chair yoga exercises are tailored to help you develop better coordination and strength, giving you the confidence to move through your daily activities safely and with ease.

Imagine being able to reach for an item on a high shelf, walk across a room, or stand up from a seated position without worrying about losing your balance. Improved stability and balance make all of these tasks, and more, much easier and safer. This chapter provides targeted chair yoga poses that are accessible and effective, allowing you to build your stability and balance gradually and safely.

Seated Chair Tree

Helps with:	
» **Muscle strengthening** It strengthens the legs and core muscles, improving overall lower body strength.	» **Improved posture** Engaging the core and maintaining alignment of the spine helps our posture.

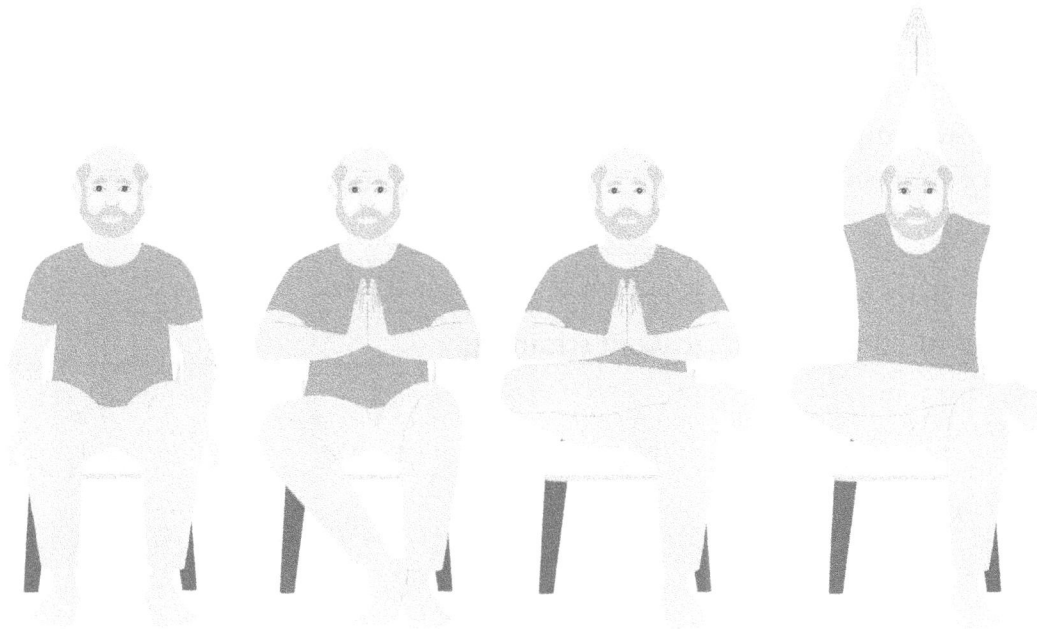

Steps:

1. Begin by sitting upright in a stable chair, with your feet firmly planted on the floor. This position ensures proper posture and balance from the start.

2. Carefully place your right foot on top of the left thigh, making sure to avoid resting it directly on the knee joint. For a less intense variation, rest your right foot on your left ankle instead.

3. Gently press your right knee towards the floor to open up the hip. This movement should be done gently to avoid strain, focusing on the stretch and opening of the hip.

4. Bring your hands together in a prayer position at your chest or, for an added challenge, raise them overhead, keeping your shoulders away from your ears. This adds an element of balance and focus to the pose.

5. Hold this position for 5-10 breaths, focusing on maintaining balance and stability. The breath will aid in concentration and steadiness.

6. After completing one side, gently release and switch sides, repeating the process with the left foot on the right thigh or ankle.

Chair Reverse Warrior

Helps with:	
» **Improved balance and coordination** This pose enhances your stability and coordination by engaging the core and leg muscles while reaching backward. » **Enhanced joint flexibility** The pose stretches the sides of the body, hips, and spine, improving joint flexibility and range of motion.	» **Muscle strengthening** It strengthens the legs, core, and arms, providing better overall body support and stability. » **Improved posture** Engaging the core and maintaining an upright position helps promote proper posture and spinal alignment.
Safety Precautions: - Ensure the chair is stable. - Be mindful of your balance to avoid straining.	

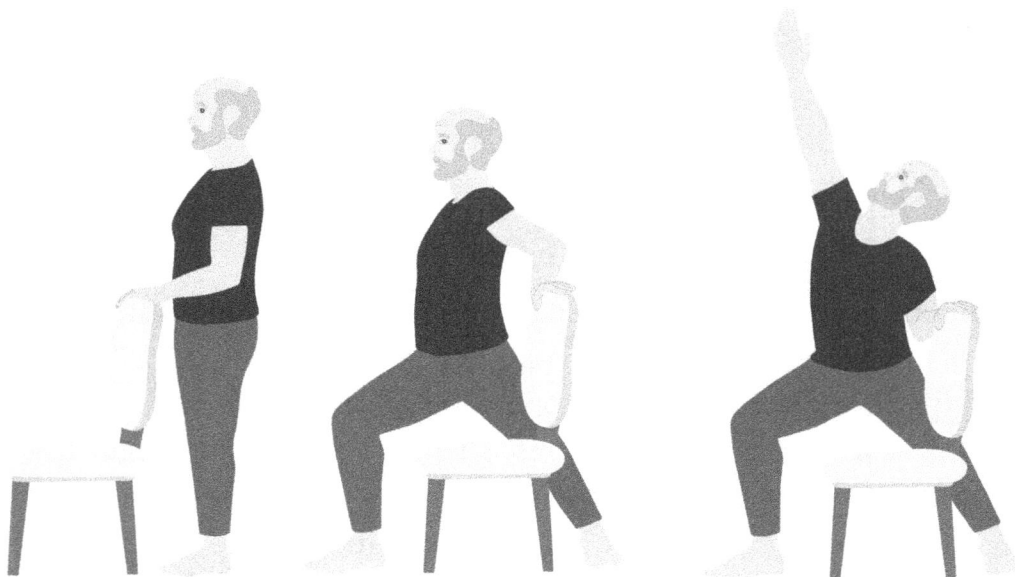

<u>Steps:</u>

1. Begin by standing to the side of the chair, with the chair on your left side for support. Grasp the back of the chair with your left hand to ensure stability throughout the pose.

2. Step your right foot forward into a lunge, bending your right knee so it aligns directly over your right ankle. Keep your left leg straight and strong, grounding through the heel.

3. Carefully lean your torso back slightly, extending your right arm up and over your head to create a gentle arc with your body. This movement stretches the side torso and engages the legs.

4. Turn your gaze upwards, looking towards your right hand. This not only enhances the stretch but also aids in improving balance and focus.

5. Maintain this pose for a few deep breaths, concentrating on the stretch and strength being cultivated in the pose.

6. To exit the pose, gently straighten your torso and release your right arm down, then step back to the starting position. Switch sides and repeat the steps with your left foot forward.

Seated High Leg Marches

Helps with:	
» **Muscle strengthening** This exercise targets the hip flexors, quadriceps, and core, building strength in the lower body. » **Improved circulation** It promotes blood flow to the lower body, improving overall circulation.	» **Improved balance and coordination** The marching motion enhances coordination and stability.
Safety Precautions:	
- Move in a controlled manner to avoid losing balance. - Suitable for those seeking a low-impact cardio exercise.	

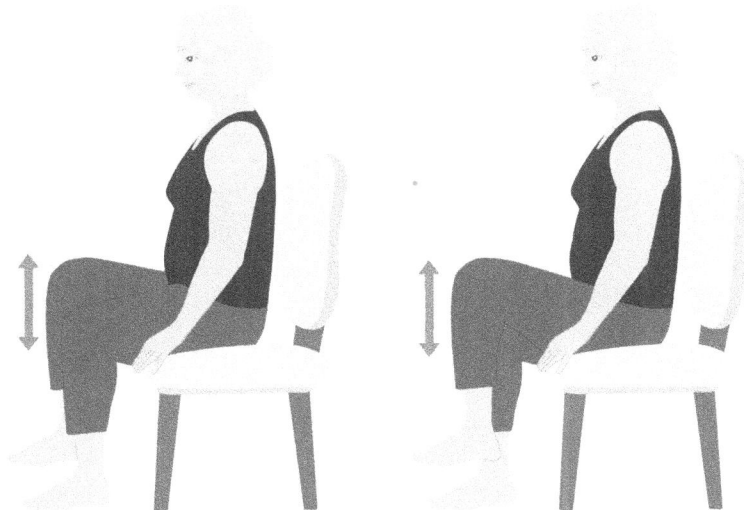

Steps:

1. Begin by sitting upright on a chair, ensuring your feet are flat on the ground. This starting position promotes good posture and stability throughout the exercise.

2. Engage your core muscles to provide additional support for your upper body. Then, lift one knee as high as comfortably possible, mimicking a marching motion. The higher you lift your knee, the more you engage the muscles in your leg and hip.

3. Lower the lifted knee back to the starting position and then lift the other knee, continuing the marching motion. This alternating action helps to evenly work both legs while also promoting coordination and balance.

4. Continue this rhythmic marching motion for 30 seconds to 1 minute, depending on your comfort and fitness level. Focus on maintaining a controlled pace to maximize the cardiovascular benefits without risking balance.

5. As you perform the exercise, breathe evenly and maintain an upright posture to ensure effective engagement of your core and leg muscles.

Seated Downward Dog

Helps with:	
» **Muscle strengthening** This pose engages the arms, shoulders, and core, building upper body strength.	» **Improved balance and coordination** Stretching and strengthening the muscles used in balance improves overall stability.
» **Improved flexibility** The pose stretches the spine and hamstrings, enhancing flexibility in these areas.	
Safety Precautions:	
- Maintain a neutral neck position. - Adjust the intensity of the stretch to avoid discomfort, especially if you have back issues.	

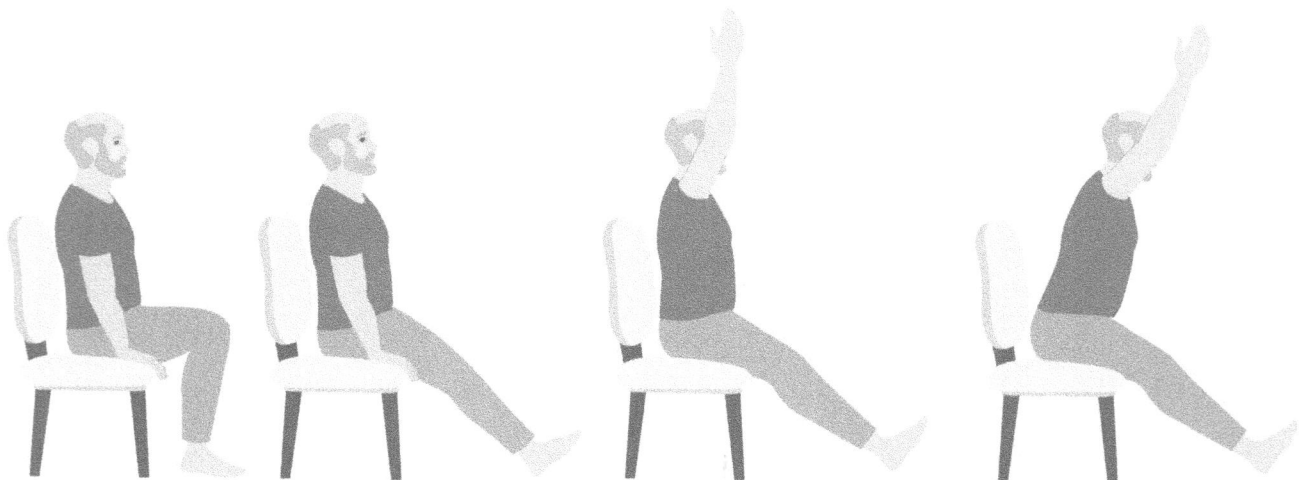

1. Begin by sitting towards the front of your chair, creating an active and alert seated posture. Extend your legs straight in front of you, resting your heels on the floor, and flexing your toes towards you. Alternatively, if it feels more comfortable, bend your knees and place your feet flat on the floor.

2. With an inhale, extend your arms straight out in front of you or alongside your ears and fold forward slightly at your hips, not from the waist, and ensure your back is completely straight. Adjust the height of your arms to what feels most sustainable.

3. Actively draw your shoulder blades down and away from your ears, creating space and reducing tension in the neck and upper back.

4. Focus your gaze downward, toward your navel or at a fixed point on the ground between your legs. This helps maintain a neutral neck position & concentration.

5. Hold this position for several deep, even breaths. With each exhale, imagine releasing tension in the spine, shoulders, and hamstrings, deepening the stretch.

6. To exit the pose, gently raise your torso back up to an upright seated position on an inhale, lowering your arms to your sides or placing them on your lap.

Seated Warrior II

Helps with:	
» **Muscle strengthening** This pose strengthens the legs, hips, and core, building overall lower body strength.	» **Improved balance and coordination** The wide stance and arm extension improve balance and stability.
» **Improved posture** Engaging the core and aligning the spine helps improve posture.	
Safety Precautions:	
- Ensure proper alignment to avoid strain. - Avoid if you have hip or knee injuries.	

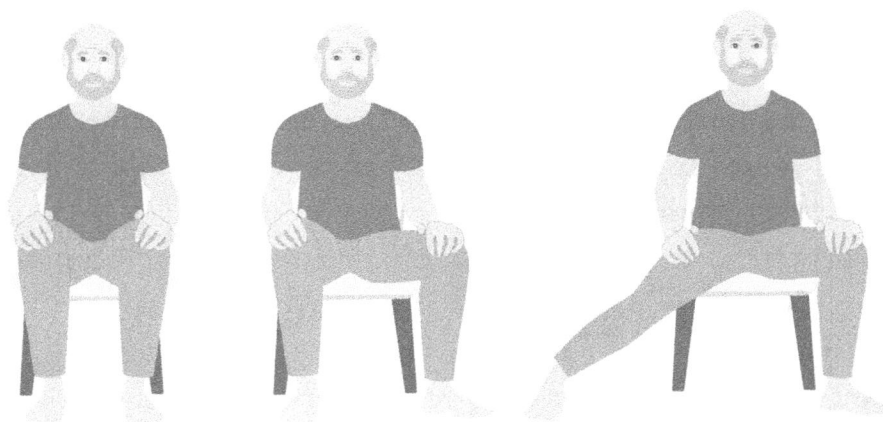

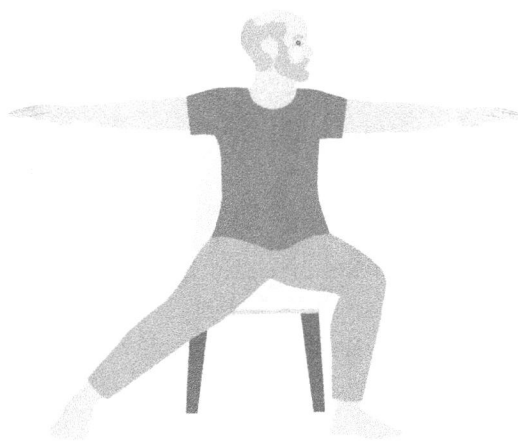

Steps:

1. Begin by sitting on the edge of a chair, ensuring your spine is erect and your hands gently rest on your knees. Your feet should be flat on the floor, spaced apart at shoulder width for a stable foundation.

2. Open your left leg to the side, creating a 90-degree angle at the knee, with your foot firmly planted and toes pointing to the left. This movement begins the process of opening up the hips and strengthening the thigh muscles.

3. Extend your right leg back, straightening the knee, and place your foot flat on the ground with your toes pointing forward. This position stretches the hip flexors and calves, contributing to the overall strengthening of the lower body.

4. Elevate your arms to shoulder height, reaching them outward to the sides in a powerful stance. This not only strengthens the arms and shoulders but also helps in maintaining balance.

5. Turn your head to gaze towards your left hand, aligning your focus with your body's direction. Hold this posture for three to four deep breaths, feeling the strength and stability in your pose.

6. To release, gently turn your head back to the center, lower your arms, and bring your legs back to the initial position. This careful, controlled movement ensures a safe and effective practice.

7. Repeat the pose on the other side: Shift your right leg to the side this time, creating a 90-degree angle at the knee, and extend your left leg back. Turn your head to gaze towards your right hand. Hold for three to four breaths before returning to the starting position.

Chair Half Moon Balance

Helps with:	
» **Improved balance and coordination** This pose enhances your sense of balance and coordination by requiring stabilization while extending one leg and one arm.	» **Myofascial Pain Syndrome** It strengthens the core, leg, and hip muscles, providing better support for your body.
» **Enhanced joint flexibility** The pose stretches the hip flexors, hamstrings, and spine, improving joint flexibility.	» **Improved posture** Engaging your core and aligning your spine in this pose promotes proper posture.
Safety Precautions:	
- Use the chair for support to maintain balance. - Avoid if you have balance or lower body mobility issues.	

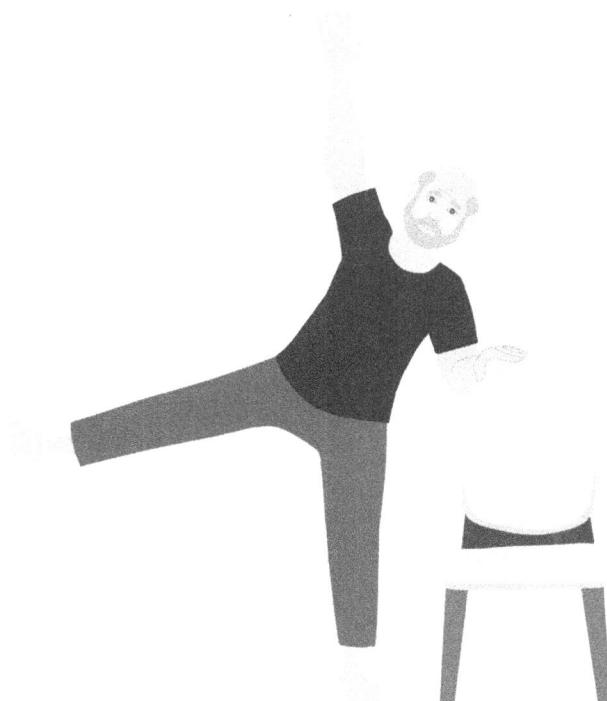

1. Begin by standing with your left side next to the chair, placing your left hand on the backrest for support. This ensures stability as you enter the pose.

2. Carefully shift your weight onto your left leg, grounding through the foot for balance. This activates the muscles in the standing leg, preparing them for the pose.

3. Gradually lift your right leg to the side, keeping it straight, while simultaneously tilting your torso to the left. Aim to create a straight line from your left foot through your torso and out through your right fingertips, which are reaching towards the sky.

4. As you balance, extend your right arm upward, directly in line with your left leg. This action not only enhances the stretch along the right side of your body but also encourages a strong sense of balance and alignment.

5. Maintain this position for a few deep, steady breaths, focusing on the stretch and strength being cultivated in the pose.

6. To exit, gently lower your right leg back to the ground and return to a standing position before switching sides to ensure a balanced practice.

Seated Crescent Lunge Pose

Helps with:	
» **Muscle strengthening** This pose challenges your balance by requiring stabilization while extending one leg behind, enhancing overall coordination.	» **Improved balance and coordination** This pose challenges your balance by requiring stabilization while extending one leg behind, enhancing overall coordination.
» **Enhanced joint flexibility** The pose stretches the hip flexors and quadriceps, increasing flexibility and range of motion in the hips and legs.	
Safety Precautions:	
- Ensure the chair is stable. - Avoid if you have severe knee or hip pain.	

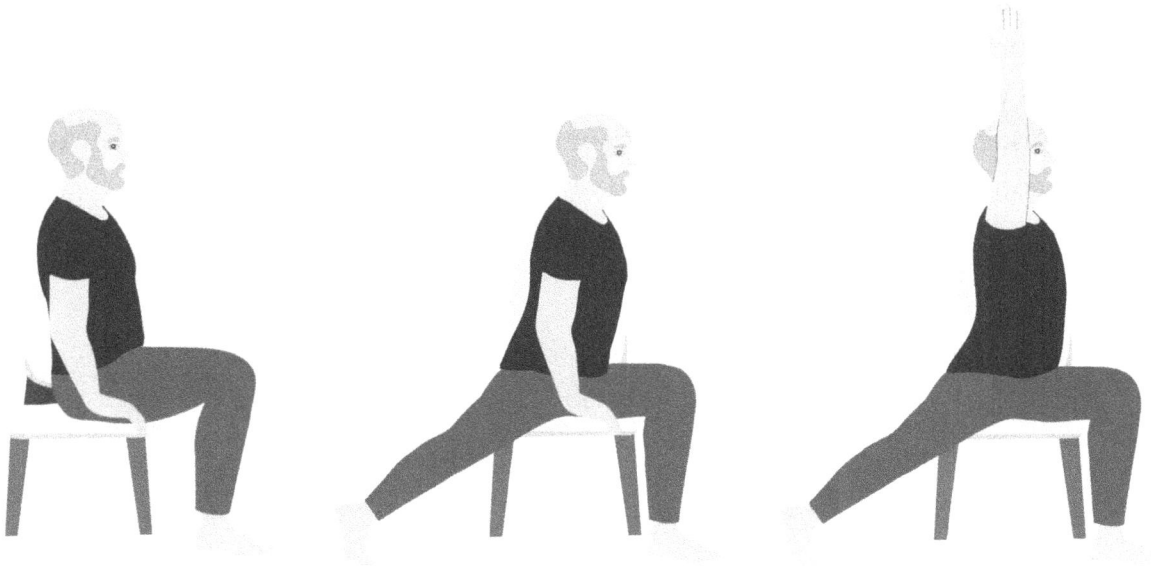

<u>Steps:</u>

1. Begin by sitting at the edge of your chair, turning your legs and body to the left side, ensuring it's stable.

2. Inhale deeply and step your right foot back into a high lunge, positioning the back heel straight up to the sky and bend your front knee to a 90-degree angle, ensuring it is directly above your ankle. This posture starts the engagement and strengthening of your legs.

3. Your back leg should be straight, with the heel lifted off the ground, mimicking the stance of a traditional Crescent Lunge. This engages the thigh muscles of your back leg for stability and a deeper stretch in the hip flexor.

4. Inhale and raise your arms above your head if balance allows, or keep your hands on the chair for support. Engage your core to keep your torso upright and stable.

5. Gently arch your back and open your chest towards the ceiling, creating a slight backbend to enhance the stretch in your chest and front body.

6. Hold the pose for several breaths, focusing on a deep stretch through the hip flexor of the back leg and maintaining balance and stability.

7. To exit the pose, carefully lower your arms (if raised) and step your back foot forward to return to your sitting position.

8. Repeat the pose with the opposite leg forward to ensure a balanced workout.

Stability and balance are vital for maintaining your independence and safety. By regularly practicing these targeted chair yoga exercises, you'll notice a significant improvement in your coordination, strength, and overall confidence. With better balance and stability, you'll reduce your risk of falls and make daily activities like walking, standing, and reaching much easier and more secure.

Incorporating these movements into your routine will not only enhance your physical health but also promote a more active and fulfilling lifestyle. You'll find yourself moving with greater ease and assurance, enjoying increased independence and a heightened sense of well-being. Let's work together to build your strength and balance, empowering you to live your daily life with confidence and capability. You've got this!

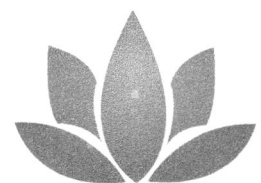

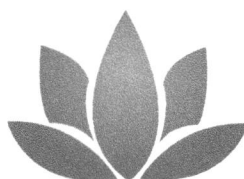

CHAPTER 8
CREATING A DAILY ROUTINE WITH CHAIR YOGA

Creating a daily routine is key, especially when it involves something as beneficial as chair yoga. In this chapter I am going to guide you and help you to integrate chair yoga into your everyday life, making it a habit that sticks and brings long-term benefits. We'll cover everything from starting with short sequences to gradually increasing the challenge, and staying motivated. Let's dive in and build a routine that enhances your physical abilities and gets your mobility skyrocketing.

IMPORTANCE OF CONSISTENCY IN PRACTICE

First off, consistency is key. Building a consistent chair yoga practice is crucial for reaping the long-term benefits. Consistency helps in forming healthy habits that are easier to maintain over time. When you practice regularly, you create a rhythm that your body and mind come to rely on, making it easier to stick with the routine.

Regular chair yoga practice leads to cumulative physical and mental health benefits. Each session builds on the previous one, gradually enhancing your strength, and flexibility, and mobility. The more consistent you are, the more pronounced these benefits become.

The mind-body connection strengthens through consistent practice. When you regularly engage in mindful movements and breathing exercises, you become more in tune with your body's signals. This heightened awareness can lead to better stress management and emotional balance.

STARTING WITH SHORT SEQUENCES

For beginners, starting with short sequences can make chair yoga feel more manageable and less overwhelming. Let's talk about a few easy ways to incorporate these short sessions into your day.

» **5-Minute Morning Routine**: Introducing a simple 5-minute morning routine can set a positive tone for the day. A quick session that includes gentle stretches and deep breathing can boost your energy and focus, making it easier to tackle daily tasks. For example, start with some seated shoulder shrugs, followed by a gentle seated forward bend, and finish with a few deep breaths to center yourself.

» **10-Minute Evening Routine**: A 10-minute evening routine can help you wind down and prepare for a restful night's sleep. Incorporating calming poses and relaxation techniques can alleviate tension and promote better sleep quality. Think about ending your day with seated cat-cow stretches, gentle neck stretches, and a seated twist to release any remaining tension.

» **Midday Stretch Breaks**: Midday stretch breaks can be a lifesaver during busy days. Short sequences that you can perform before or after lunch or between tasks can refresh your mind and body, reducing fatigue and improving energy levels. Simple moves like seated side bends, seated chest openers, and seated spinal twists can keep you feeling flexible and focused throughout the day.

GRADUAL PROGRESSION AND INCREASING CHALLENGE

Listening to your body is crucial when practicing chair yoga. Pay attention to how you feel during and after each session. Progress at your own pace, and don't push yourself too hard. The goal is to gradually build strength and flexibility without causing injury.

» **Incremental Time Increase**: Start with short sessions and gradually increase the duration of your practice. Begin with 5-minute sessions and slowly work your way up to 15, 20, and eventually 30 minutes as you become more comfortable and confident. This incremental approach allows your body to adapt and grow stronger over time.

» **Adding New Poses**: As your strength and flexibility improve, start incorporating new and slightly more challenging poses. This gradual introduction of new poses keeps your practice engaging and helps you progress safely. For example, you might start with seated calf raises and progress to seated warrior poses as your balance and strength improve.

» **Incorporating Variations**: Variations of basic poses can increase the difficulty and engage different muscle groups. Adding these variations to your routine can help you build strength and flexibility in a balanced way. For instance, you can modify a seated forward bend by adding a twist or extending one leg at a time to target different areas of your body.

YOUR FLEXIBLE CHAIR YOGA ROUTINE FOR MOBILITY WEEKLY PLAN SAMPLE

To help you get started, here is a sample weekly routine plan. This plan is designed to be flexible, allowing you to easily adjust and change the exercises based on which areas you want to focus.

Instructions:

1. **Begin each day with a breathing technique and some warm-up exercises.** This will help to center your mind and prepare your body for the chair yoga session.

2. **Follow the sequence of poses as outlined for each day.** Hold each pose for 30 - 45 seconds based on how you feel.

3. **Take a short pause of 15 seconds between each exercise or pose.** Use this time to breathe normally and prepare for the next pose.

4. **Remember to go at your own pace.** It's important to listen to your body and not push beyond comfort. If you experience any discomfort, modify the pose or skip it as needed.

5. **Begin with the goal of practicing these chair yoga workouts daily.** I know that you're busy, but I've found that this consistent approach helps students to establish a routine and maximize the benefits of the program.
    » However, it's important to listen to your body and be mindful of your energy levels and physical comfort.
    » If you find that daily practice is too demanding, or if you experience any discomfort, it's perfectly fine to adjust your schedule.
    » In such cases, aim to complete the workouts 4 to 5 times a week instead.
    » This adjustment ensures that you still maintain regular practice while giving your body adequate time to rest and recover.

I'm here to support you on your journey to a healthier, happier life. If you have any questions, concerns, or would like a few words of encouragement, please don't hesitate to reach out (jcharrisonbooks@gmail.com).

Here is an example of what doing some exercises from Part I - chapter 4 might look like.

WEEK 1 SAMPLE ROUTINE FOR MOBILITY		
Box Breathing (perform for 30-45s, page 22)		
INHALE 4 SECONDS · HOLD 4 SECONDS · EXHALE 4 SECONDS · HOLD 4 SECONDS		
Ankle and Wrist Rotations (30-45s, page 31)	Torso Twists (30-45s, page 30)	Shoulder Rolls (30-45s, page 36)
Seated Spinal Twist (30-45s, page 33)	Chair Cat-Cow Stretch (30-45s, page 34)	Seated Forward Bend (30-45s, page 35)
Remember to take a short pause of 15 seconds between each exercise or pose.		

For week 2 feel free to try some of the other exercises from Chapter 4 or you can do exercises from a different chapter to target another pain point in your body.

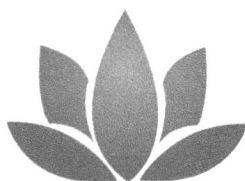

CONCLUSION

As we reach the end of this book, let's take a moment to reflect on the journey we've embarked upon together. Chair yoga has proven itself to be a remarkable tool for enhancing mobility and flexibility, particularly for seniors. We've explored exercises designed to improve joint health, build muscle strength and elasticity, reduce pain and tension, and enhance stability and balance. Each chapter has equipped you with practical, accessible techniques to support your overall well-being and empower you to lead a more active and fulfilling life.

Now, it's time to take everything you've learned and make it a part of your daily routine. The benefits of chair yoga extend far beyond the immediate relief you might feel after a session. With consistent practice, you will experience lasting improvements in your mobility, flexibility, strength, and balance. More importantly, you'll find that your overall sense of well-being improves. Your commitment to this practice will reward you with a healthier, more vibrant life. So, keep pushing yourself, stay dedicated, and remember that every stretch, every pose, brings you closer to your goals.

To keep your momentum going, set personal goals for your chair yoga journey. Whether it's increasing your flexibility, alleviating chronic pain, or enhancing your balance, having clear targets will keep you motivated and focused. Track your progress along the way. Celebrate your successes, no matter how small they might seem. Each step forward is a victory, a testament to your dedication and hard work. By documenting your journey, you'll have a powerful reminder of how far you've come and the amazing progress you've made.

Remember, true health is about more than just physical fitness. It's about nurturing your mind, body, and spirit. Chair yoga offers a holistic approach to health and aging, addressing all these aspects. As you continue your practice, embrace this interconnectedness. Use your time on the mat to cultivate not only your physical strength and flexibility but also your mental clarity and emotional resilience. This comprehensive approach will enrich your life in ways that go beyond the physical, helping you achieve a balanced, fulfilling lifestyle.

Congratulations on completing this journey through chair yoga. Your commitment to improving your health and well-being is truly inspiring. Keep pushing yourself, stay motivated, and never underestimate the power of your efforts. Every stretch, every breath, every moment you dedicate to your practice brings you closer to a more active, independent, and joyful life. You have the tools, the knowledge, and the strength within you to continue this journey. Embrace it fully, and let the benefits of chair yoga empower you to live your best life.

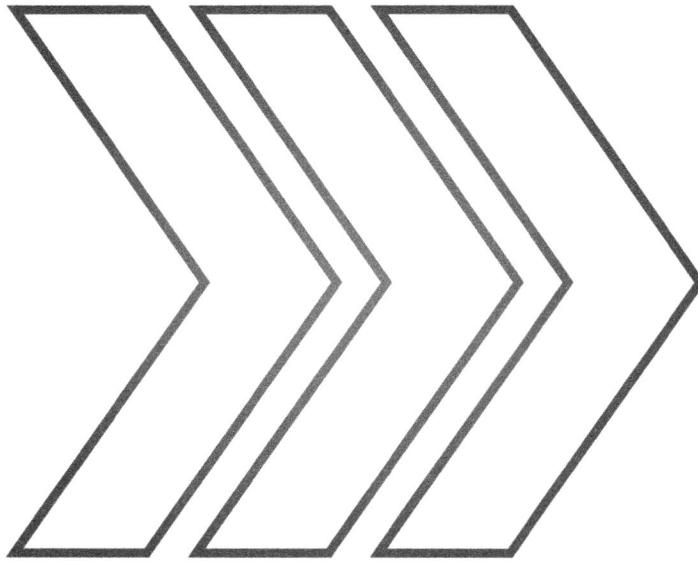

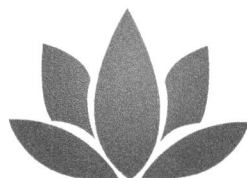

PART II
CHAIR YOGA FOR SENIORS PAIN MANAGEMENT

Low Impact, Easy To Follow Seated Exercises To Help Manage Arthritis, Fibromyalgia, Back Aches, Shoulder Discomfort, Neck Stiffness, Inflammation and all Types of Chronic Pain.

J.C. Harrison

Gran Publications

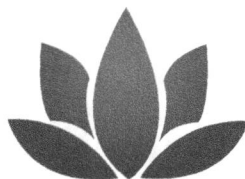

INTRODUCTION

Imagine a time when getting out of bed was effortless, a time when you could move freely without a second thought. Remember the joy of kneeling down to tend your garden, strolling through the park with ease, or playing with your grandchildren without a hint of discomfort. Those moments of pure freedom and joy now seem like distant memories as chronic pain and stiffness have taken over. It's that lingering discomfort that can put a damper on your favorite activities, disrupt your sleep, and make even the simplest tasks feel daunting.

Pain is a reality for many seniors, but that doesn't mean it has to control your life. The search for effective pain management solutions is not just about finding temporary relief; it's about reclaiming your independence and enjoying your golden years to the fullest. This book is here to introduce you to a practice that will change everything for you: Chair Yoga For Seniors Pain Management.

My name is JC Harrison, and I've dedicated my life to helping seniors reclaim their mobility, independence, and joy through chair yoga. Inspired by my own mother's journey to maintain her fitness and health as she grew older, I created a comprehensive chair yoga program tailored specifically for seniors. With years of experience in senior fitness and wellness, I help seniors become pain-free, increase their mobility, and regain their independence, all from the comfort of their chair!

Chair yoga offers a gentle yet powerful approach to pain management, providing seniors with a safe and accessible way to improve flexibility, reduce discomfort, and enhance overall well-being. Unlike traditional yoga, chair yoga adapts poses so they can be performed while seated or using the chair for support, making it perfect for those with chronic pain or mobility issues. You don't need to be an expert or have any prior experience with yoga to benefit from chair yoga. All you need is a chair and a willingness to try something new.

By incorporating simple chair yoga techniques into your daily routine, you can experience increased comfort and mobility in your everyday life. Imagine being able to move with greater ease, bending down without wincing, and feeling more confident in your body's abilities. Chair yoga not only addresses physical pain but also promotes mental relaxation and emotional well-being. It provides a holistic way to care for your body and mind.

In this book, we will delve into the fundamentals of chair yoga for pain management, guiding you through essential techniques and exercises designed specifically for seniors. We'll start with setting up your practice space, ensuring you have everything you need to create a comfortable and supportive environment. From there, we'll explore various chair yoga poses that target areas commonly affected by pain, such as the back, shoulders, hips, and legs. Each chapter will offer step-by-step instructions, accompanied by illustrations to help you perform the poses correctly and safely.

As you progress through the chapters, you'll find tips on how to adapt the poses to suit your individual needs and limitations. Whether you're dealing with arthritis, recovering from surgery, or simply wanting to improve your overall mobility, there's something in this book for everyone. You'll also discover breathing exercises and mindfulness techniques that complement the physical practice of chair yoga, enhancing its benefits and helping you achieve a deeper sense of relaxation and presence.

By the end of this book, you will have a comprehensive understanding of how chair yoga can be integrated into your daily routine, empowering you to take charge of your health and well-being. You'll learn how to listen to your body, honor its limits, and celebrate its strengths. Chair yoga isn't just a series of exercises; it's a journey of self-discovery and self-care, offering you the opportunity to connect with yourself in a meaningful way.

Embracing chair yoga as a daily practice means prioritizing your health and well-being. It's about taking proactive steps to alleviate discomfort and enhance your quality of life. With dedication and consistency, you have the power to transform how you experience pain, shifting from a state of dependency and frustration to one of empowerment and resilience. By investing time in your practice, you're investing in yourself, and that's a decision you'll never regret.

So, let's embark on this journey together. Let's explore the wonderful world of chair yoga and uncover the many ways it can enrich your life. In the coming chapters, you'll find the knowledge, tools, and inspiration needed to make chair yoga a regular part of your routine. Whether you're new to yoga or a seasoned practitioner looking for a gentler approach, this book will provide you with everything you need to get started and stay motivated.

Remember, managing pain doesn't have to be an uphill battle. With chair yoga, you have a valuable ally on your side. It's time to take control of your well-being, embrace this transformative practice, and start living life with greater ease and joy. Welcome to the beginning of a new chapter in your journey towards better health and happiness.

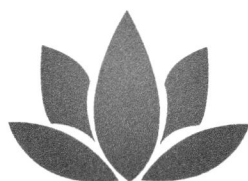

CHAPTER 1
CHAIR YOGA FOR PAIN MANAGEMENT

Chair yoga is a game-changer for seniors dealing with pain. Instead of struggling to get up and down from the floor, chair yoga uses a chair for support, allowing you to perform controlled stretches and strengthening exercises without overexertion.

In this chapter, we'll dive into the essentials of chair yoga and why it's a must for seniors managing pain. Discover how chair yoga modifies traditional poses to be performed while seated, ensuring safety and accessibility. Learn about the inclusivity of chair yoga, designed for conditions like arthritis, joint pain, and muscle stiffness. Explore the broad range of motions in chair yoga, such as neck rolls, seated twists, and forward bends, which are crucial for maintaining flexibility, mobility, and a pain-free life. We'll also discuss the mental relaxation techniques that often accompany chair yoga, contributing to emotional well-being and stress reduction. Finally, find out how props like chairs, straps, and blocks can enhance the overall chair yoga experience, making it adaptable to individual needs and limitations.

WHAT IS CHAIR YOGA AND WHY DOES IT WORK SO WELL AT FIGHTING PAIN?

What is Chair Yoga exactly? Chair yoga takes traditional yoga poses and modifies them into a seated format, making it highly suitable for seniors. Traditional yoga demands significant mobility and balance, often excluding older adults with physical limitations. Chair yoga changes the game by allowing these poses to be done while sitting, providing a safe, accessible way for seniors to engage in yoga without extensive physical exertion or balance requirements. Using a chair for support, seniors can effectively perform stretches and strengthening exercises, experiencing the benefits of yoga in a more controlled and less intimidating environment.

Inclusivity is a key aspect of chair yoga. For seniors facing challenges such as arthritis, joint pain, or muscle stiffness, getting down on the floor and back up again can be daunting, sometimes impossible. Chair yoga removes this barrier by ensuring most movements are performed while seated, opening the world of yoga to those who might otherwise be unable to participate. This adaptation not only increases accessibility but also decreases the risk of injury, offering a comforting and secure alternative to traditional yoga practices.

The chair yoga poses I have designed for this book typically incorporate a wide range of motions that mimic regular yoga activities. Each of these movements helps maintain flexibility and mobility, which are crucial for day-to-day pain-free functioning and independence among seniors. The ability to sustain such physical activity without risking falls or overexertion makes my chair yoga program a preferred choice for elderly participants.

These poses offer substantial benefits not only for pain mangement but also for enhancing flexibility, strength, and overall well-being in older adults. Flexibility tends to decrease with age, leading to stiffness and reduced mobility, which can significantly impact an individual's quality of life. Chair yoga focuses on gently stretching various muscle groups, enhancing joint health, and maintaining muscle elasticity. Over time, this can lead to improved range of motion and decreased stiffness, supporting daily activities like bending, reaching, and walking.

Strengthening exercises are another cornerstone of chair yoga. While seated, participants engage in muscle-strengthening poses that involve holding positions or using body weight for resistance. These exercises help build muscle mass and endurance, critical factors in preventing falls and maintaining independence. Stronger muscles mean better support for joints, reducing pain associated with conditions like osteoarthritis and rheumatoid arthritis. Additionally, regular practice can improve posture, further alleviating discomfort and promoting better body alignment.

Beyond physical improvements, chair yoga combines physical exercise with mental relaxation techniques. Many chair yoga routines incorporate breathing exercises and mindfulness practices that reduce stress and anxiety. These techniques enhance mental clarity and emotional stability, contributing positively to overall quality of life. Regular engagement in chair yoga fosters a harmonious balance between mind and body, aiding in pain management.

It's no secret that pain and mobility issues tend to go hand in hand. Unlike more intense forms of exercise that may exacerbate existing conditions or cause new injuries, chair yoga emphasizes slow, deliberate movements that prioritize safety. Seniors with debilitating conditions like spinal stenosis, fibromyalgia, or sciatica often find relief in the low-impact nature of chair yoga routines, minimizing strain on the body while providing therapeutic benefits.

The gentle movements in my chair yoga program accommodate varying levels of physical ability, ensuring you do not push beyond your limits. This aspect is crucial for people who might fear overstraining themselves and worsening their symptoms. With chair yoga, you can engage in a manageable workout that fits your comfort level and progressively build strength and flexibility over time. This gradual improvement encourages more consistant participation and creates more long-term health benefits for you. It's a win win!

REDUCE AND REMOVE PAIN: WHAT ELSE CAN CHAIR YOGA DO FOR YOU?

Yoga is a powerhouse for health and for seniors managing pain, by offering a gentle yet effective way to maintain and even improve overall well-being, keeping you strong, balanced, and mentally sharp.

One primary advantage of yoga for seniors is its ability to enhance balance, flexibility, and posture. As we age, these physical attributes become crucial. Yoga poses like tree pose or seated forward bend stretch and strengthen muscles, making you feel more stable and secure in your movements. Improved balance slashes the risk of falls, a huge concern for older adults. Flexibility gained through regular practice alleviates stiffness, making everyday tasks easier and less painful.

Yoga also promotes better posture. Many seniors struggle with poor posture due to years of sedentary behavior or muscle weakness. Yoga encourages alignment and proper body mechanics, preventing chronic conditions like rounded shoulders or kyphosis. Poses that open the chest and strengthen back muscles help you maintain a tall, upright posture, boosting confidence and comfort.

The mental benefits of yoga are just as significant. Stress reduction is a top perk, especially for seniors facing anxiety related to health concerns or life changes. Deep breathing techniques practiced in yoga activate your body's relaxation response, lowering cortisol levels and promoting a sense of calm and tranquility. This stress relief can lead to lower blood pressure and better heart health.

Improved focus and cognitive function are additional mental benefits. Seniors engaging in mindful movement and meditation often find their attention span and memory improves, helping you hold on to those precious memories just a little longer. Concentrating on holding poses and coordinating breath with movement sharpens the mind, offering a natural way to combat age-related cognitive decline. And with enhanced mental clarity, that makes daily activities more manageable and enjoyable.

Yoga's emphasis on mindfulness and being present supports emotional well-being. Seniors practicing yoga report feeling more connected to their bodies and emotions, leading to greater self-awareness and a positive outlook on life. This holistic approach fosters mental resilience, helping you cope better with the challenges of aging.

THE PAIN-FREE PROMISE OF CHAIR YOGA: WHAT YOU NEED TO KNOW

Chair yoga has been a proven asset for seniors battling chronic pain. By adapting traditional yoga poses into a seated format, it cuts the risk associated with more strenuous forms of exercise, making it accessible for those with conditions like osteoarthritis or degenerative disc disease. Seniors can find relief from various types of chronic pain, including back pain and arthritis. Gentle stretching and strengthening exercises boost joint flexibility and reduce stiffness, offering significant pain relief.

Take lower back pain, for example. Many seniors I have worked with suffer from it due to degenerative disc disease or sciatica. Chair yoga incorporates specific stretches targeting the lumbar region, helping to alleviate tension and improve spinal alignment. Regular practice can reduce inflammation and muscle spasms, decreasing overall discomfort. For those with arthritis in their knees or hips, chair yoga provides exercises to strengthen surrounding muscles, improving joint stability and cutting down on pain during movement.

Chair yoga also enhances mobility and range of motion. As we age, our joints get stiffer, leading to decreased movement and a higher risk of falls. Techniques like modified sun salutations and seated twists gently stretch and lubricate the joints, increasing flexibility. Better joint health translates to improved balance and coordination, crucial for daily activities. Regular engagement in these exercises helps you regain lost mobility, allowing them to move more freely and confidently.

Strengthening muscles around critical joints, such as the knees and hips, is another huge benefit of regular chair yoga practice. Stronger muscles provide better support and reduce the load on affected joints, which is particularly beneficial for those with osteoarthritis. Over time, increased muscle support improves walking ability and reduces reliance on assistive devices. Enhanced mobility not only makes physical activities easier but also encourages an active lifestyle, vital for overall health.

The mind-body connection fostered by yoga is powerful. Chair yoga emphasizes mindful movement and conscious breathing, increasing body awareness. For seniors managing chronic pain, becoming more attuned to their bodies can significantly impact how they perceive and manage pain. Techniques like deep breathing and guided relaxation activate the parasympathetic nervous system, promoting relaxation and reducing stress levels. This holistic approach helps break the cycle of pain, anxiety, and tension often experienced by those with chronic conditions.

Mindfulness practices incorporated into chair yoga sessions enhance emotional well-being. Many seniors face mental health challenges like depression and anxiety, often worsened by chronic pain. Focused breathing and meditation offer effective tools to manage these symptoms. Increased body awareness and relaxation techniques create a sense of peace and calm, reducing the psychological impact of chronic pain. This comprehensive approach addresses both physical and emotional aspects of well-being, making chair yoga a valuable tool in pain management.

Ultimately, chair yoga can significantly improve the overall quality of life for seniors. By reducing pain and promoting well-being, seniors can engage more fully in their daily activities and enjoy greater independence. Chronic pain often limits social interaction and participation in community events. Alleviating pain through chair yoga opens opportunities for seniors to reconnect with friends and family, enhancing their social lives and emotional health.

YOUR BLUEPRINT FOR PAIN-FREE LIVING

Managing pain is vital for seniors, especially those dealing with chronic conditions like back pain, arthritis, neck pain, shoulder pain, and muscle stiffness. Each type of pain presents unique challenges that can seriously mess with your daily routine. Back pain from issues like degenerative disc disease or sciatica can limit your mobility, making simple tasks like bending or lifting a nightmare. Joint and arthritis pain, including osteoarthritis and rheumatoid arthritis, cause severe discomfort in your knees, hips, and other joints, leading to swelling and stiffness. Neck pain from cervical spondylosis or muscle strains can give you headaches and make turning your head a struggle. Shoulder pain from rotator cuff injuries or bursitis makes reaching overhead or carrying items a hassle. Muscle stiffness from conditions like fibromyalgia creates pain throughout your body, messing with your overall flexibility and movement.

Traditionally, managing pain involves medication and physical therapy. Medications like NSAIDs, acetaminophen, and opioids can help reduce inflammation and alleviate pain, but long-term use can lead to nasty side effects and dependency, which is a big concern for older adults. Physical therapy aims to strengthen muscles, improve mobility, and reduce pain through guided exercises and stretches. While effective, physical therapy requires regular sessions and might not always be accessible or feasible for everyone.

Other methods include lifestyle changes like weight management and dietary adjustments to reduce joint stress and improve overall health. Assistive devices like walkers or braces provide support and stability. These traditional methods offer relief, but they can fall short when used in isolation.

Enter complementary therapies like yoga. Chair yoga, in particular, is a game-changer for seniors who can't perform traditional standing yoga poses due to balance issues or limited mobility. By adapting yoga postures to be performed while seated or using a chair for support, chair yoga makes the practice accessible to everyone.

Adding chair yoga to your pain management plan offers serious benefits. Gentle stretching and strengthening exercises help relieve tension and improve flexibility without putting undue strain on your joints. Deep breathing and relaxation techniques during chair yoga sessions reduce stress and anxiety, which are common in individuals dealing with chronic pain. This holistic approach ensures that both the physical and mental aspects of pain are addressed, promoting overall well-being.

Chair yoga is non-invasive and safe, making it an excellent alternative to medication and invasive procedures. It allows you to engage in physical activity at your own pace, reducing the likelihood of injury or worsening existing conditions. The low-impact nature of chair yoga makes it suitable for those with severe pain or limited mobility, ensuring everyone can participate regardless of their physical limitations.

Research backs up the positive impact of chair yoga on pain management. Studies show that chair yoga can lead to reductions in pain and improvements in physical function among older adults. Participants in chair yoga programs often report decreased pain interference in daily activities and an enhanced quality of life. By incorporating chair yoga into your routine, you can experience greater independence and a better sense of control over your pain.

Working with healthcare providers to integrate chair yoga into a comprehensive pain management strategy is crucial. Collaboration between yoga instructors, physicians, and physical therapists ensures that the practice is tailored to your individual needs and medical conditions. Healthcare providers can guide you on the appropriate intensity and frequency of chair yoga sessions, helping you maximize benefits while minimizing risks. They can also monitor your progress and make adjustments as needed, ensuring that the practice continues to meet your evolving needs.

Take control of your pain management with chair yoga. It's time to embrace a holistic, effective approach that promotes your overall well-being and helps you live your best life.

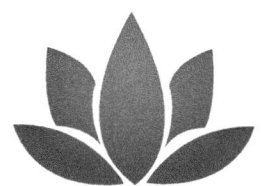

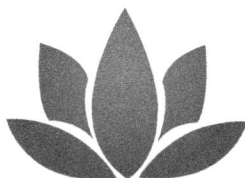

CHAPTER 2
CHAIR YOGA FOR BACK PAIN RELIEF

Let's get back to it! Back pain is a huge issue for many seniors, and it's no surprise considering the years of wear and tear our bodies endure. Conditions like degenerative disc disease, osteoarthritis, spinal stenosis, and sciatica can leave you feeling stiff, sore, and sometimes even helpless. But don't worry, this chapter is here to help. We're diving into some foundational chair yoga exercises that are simple, safe, and super effective at relieving back pain.

These chair yoga poses can target the specific types of back pain you might be dealing with:

» **Degenerative Disc Disease**: This condition can cause chronic pain and stiffness in your back. The poses we'll cover can help improve spinal flexibility and strengthen the muscles around your spine, providing much-needed support and relief.

» **Osteoarthritis**: Joint pain and stiffness from osteoarthritis can make movement difficult. Our chair yoga exercises are designed to gently stretch and strengthen your muscles, helping to ease the pressure on your joints and improve your overall mobility.

» **Spinal Stenosis**: When the spaces within your spine narrow, it can put pressure on your nerves and cause pain. The gentle movements in these poses can help increase the space in your spinal canal, reducing nerve compression and alleviating pain.

» **Sciatica**: Pain radiating down your leg from sciatica can be debilitating. Our targeted stretches can help release tension in the lower back and hips, providing relief from sciatic pain.

These exercises will help you reduce pain, improve spinal mobility, and increase overall body awareness. Let's get you moving and feeling better!

Seated Spinal Extension

Helps with:	
» **Osteoarthritis** This pose gently stretches the spine, helping to lubricate the spinal joints and reduce stiffness.	» **Degenerative Disc Disease** It increases space between the vertebrae, relieving pressure on the discs and promoting better spinal alignment.
» **Spinal Stenosis** The extending of the spine helps open up the spinal canal, reducing pressure on the spinal cord and nerves.	» **Sciatica** Stretching the spine can alleviate pressure on the sciatic nerve, reducing pain and discomfort in the lower back and legs.
Safety Precautions:	
- Do not overextend your back. - Move into the position slowly and smoothly.	

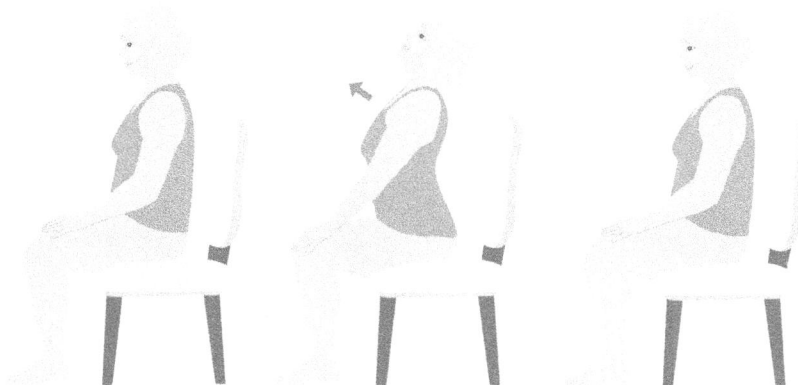

Steps:

1. Sit at the edge of a stable chair with your feet firmly planted on the ground. This starting position ensures a solid foundation for the exercise.
2. Place your hands on your thighs for support. This helps maintain balance and alignment as you move through the spinal extension.
3. Inhale deeply and gently begin to arch your back. Push your chest forward and draw your shoulders back, engaging the muscles along your spine.

4. Hold this arched position for a few seconds, allowing your back muscles to stretch and strengthen. Be mindful not to overextend; the movement should be comfortable and controlled.

5. Exhale slowly and return to your starting position, feeling the length and relaxation in your spine.

6. Repeat the exercise 5-7 times, focusing on smooth, deliberate movements. Each repetition will contribute to a greater sense of strength and flexibility in your back.

Seated Forward Fold

Helps with:	
» **Osteoarthritis** This pose stretches the lower back and hips, improving flexibility and reducing joint pain.	» **Degenerative Disc Disease** It gently decompresses the spine, providing relief from disc-related pain. » **Sciatica** By stretching the hamstrings and lower back, it helps reduce tension on the sciatic nerve, alleviating pain.
Safety Precautions:	
- Bend from your hips, not your waist. Start the movement at your hip joint, where your thigh meets your pelvis. - Avoid if you have severe lower back issues.	

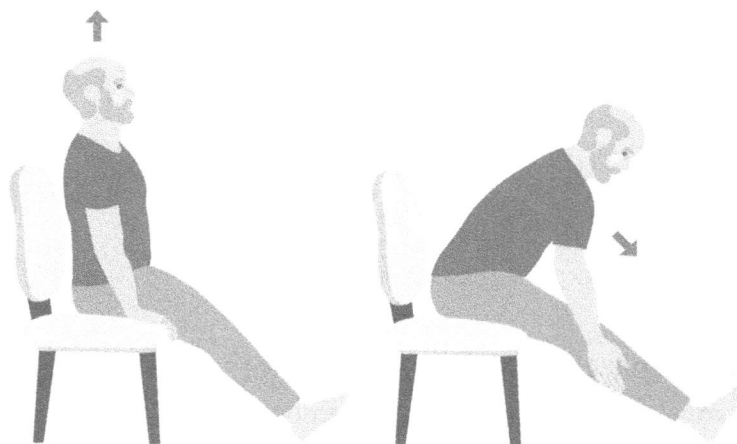

Steps:

1. Begin by sitting upright, legs extended before you, with feet positioned hip-width apart. Let this be your foundation of stability and balance.

2. Inhale deeply, inviting length into your spine, envisioning each vertebra stretching towards the sky.

3. On your exhale, pivot gracefully from your hips (to bend from the hips push your hips back while keeping your spine long and chest open), folding forward as if reaching for a moment of tranquility. Extend your hands towards your feet, embodying the gentle embrace of calm.

4. Hold this forward embrace for several nurturing breaths, allowing tension to melt away with each exhale.

5. To conclude, slowly ascend back to an upright position, carrying with you the peace and stretch you've cultivated.

Seated Side Stretch

Helps with:	
» **Osteoarthritis** This pose increases flexibility in the spine and ribcage, helping to reduce stiffness and improve range of motion. » **Spinal Stenosis** It opens up the spinal canal by stretching the side muscles, reducing nerve compression and pain.	» **Degenerative Disc Disease** Stretching the sides of the body helps create space between the vertebrae, relieving pressure on the discs.
Safety Precautions:	
- Stretch only as far as comfortable. - Avoid this exercise if you have severe rib or spine issues.	

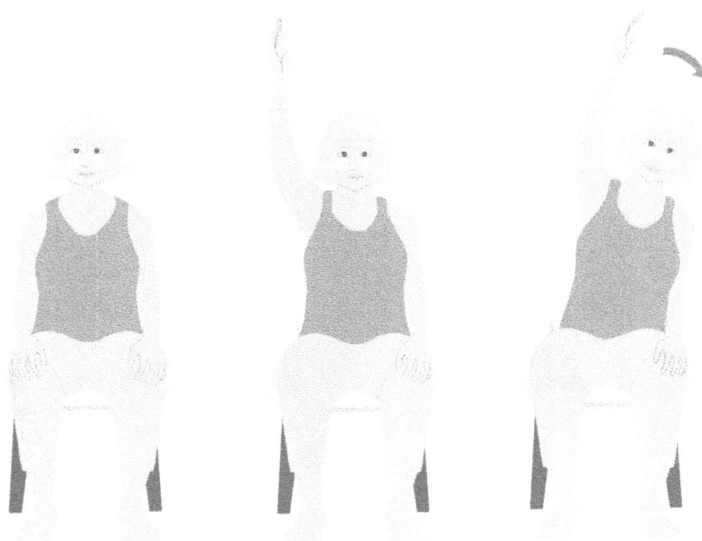

1. Start by sitting upright in a chair with your feet flat on the ground, establishing a stable and comfortable base.

2. Inhale and raise your right arm overhead, ensuring your posture remains straight and aligned.

3. As you exhale, gently lean to the left. This movement stretches the right side of your body, from the ribcage to the obliques. Move into the stretch only as far as feels comfortable, avoiding any strain.

4. Hold the position for a few breaths, allowing the stretch to deepen with each exhale. This not only enhances the stretch but also aids in relaxation.

5. Slowly return to the center and lower your arm. Then, repeat the stretch on the left side, raising your left arm and leaning to the right.

Seated Revolved Head to Knee Pose

Helps with:	
» **Osteoarthritis** It gently stretches the spine, improving flexibility and reducing stiffness. It also helps alleviate pain by increasing blood circulation and reducing inflammation.	» **Degenerative Disc Disease** By lengthening and twisting the spine, it helps create space between the vertebrae, reducing pressure on the discs.
» **Spinal Stenosis** The gentle twisting motion opens up the spinal canal, reducing compression on the spinal cord and nerves.	» **Sciatica** By stretching the hamstrings and lower back, it helps reduce tension on the sciatic nerve, alleviating pain.
Safety Precautions:	
- Stretch gently without straining. - If you have hip or hamstring issues, moderate the stretch.	

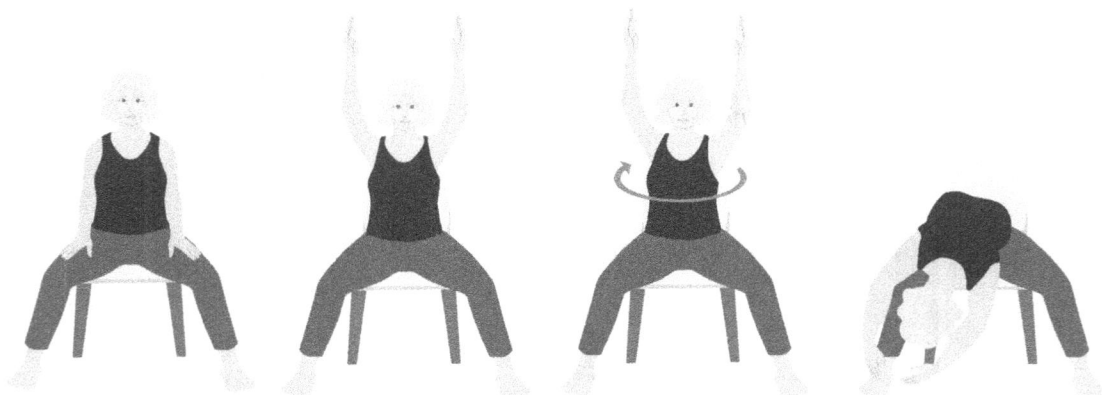

Steps:

1. Begin by sitting on a chair or a stable surface, with your legs extended wide apart in front of you. This position allows for a deep stretch without putting strain on your lower back.
2. Gently turn your torso towards your right leg, preparing your body for the side stretch. This rotation starts the engagement of your side torso muscles.
3. Inhale deeply and raise both arms overhead, creating length in your spine and preparing for the stretch. As you exhale, lean towards your right foot, extending your arms as if trying to reach your toes. Keep both arms extended to maximize the stretch along your side body.
4. Hold this position for several deep breaths, focusing on the stretch along your right side. The holding phase allows your muscles to gently elongate and relax, enhancing flexibility.
5. To come out of the pose, inhale and slowly lift your torso, bringing your arms back overhead. Then, gently turn your torso back to center and prepare to repeat the stretch on the opposite side, targeting your left leg.

Chair Cat-Cow Stretch

Helps with:	
» **Osteoarthritis** This dynamic movement increases flexibility in the spine, reducing stiffness and improving mobility.	» **Degenerative Disc Disease** Alternating between flexion and extension helps maintain disc health by promoting spinal fluid movement.
» **Spinal Stenosis** The flexing and extending of the spine can help open the spinal canal, reducing nerve compression.	» **Sciatica** This pose helps alleviate lower back tension, which can reduce pressure on the sciatic nerve.
Safety Precautions:	
- Move slowly and gently to avoid any strain. - If you have severe back pain or a spinal injury, consult with a healthcare provider before attempting this exercise.	

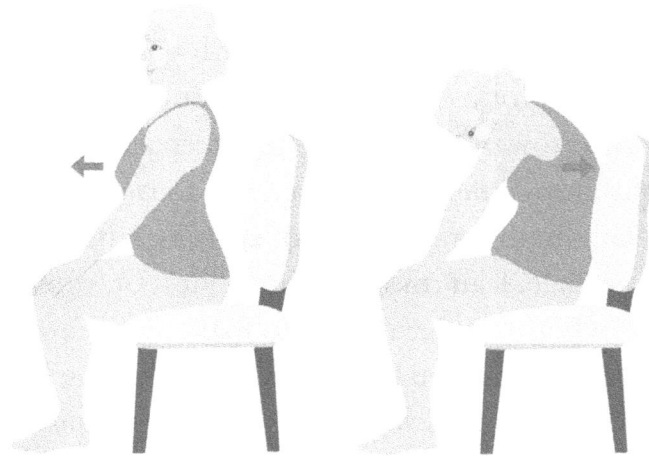

1. Begin by sitting on a chair or a stable surface, with your legs extended wide apart in front of you. This position allows for a deep stretch without putting strain on your lower back.
2. Gently turn your torso towards your right leg, preparing your body for the side stretch. This rotation starts the engagement of your side torso muscles.
3. Inhale deeply and raise both arms overhead, creating length in your spine and preparing for the stretch. As you exhale, lean towards your right foot, extending your arms as if trying to reach your toes. Keep both arms extended to maximize the stretch along your side body.
4. Hold this position for several deep breaths, focusing on the stretch along your right side. The holding phase allows your muscles to gently elongate and relax, enhancing flexibility.
5. To come out of the pose, inhale and slowly lift your torso, bringing your arms back overhead. Then, gently turn your torso back to center and prepare to repeat the stretch on the opposite side, targeting your left leg.

Seated Warrior I with Prayer Hands

Helps with:	
» **Osteoarthritis** This pose strengthens and stretches the legs and hips, reducing joint pain and improving stability.	» **Degenerative Disc Disease** It encourages good spinal alignment and strengthens the core muscles, supporting spinal health.
» **Spinal Stenosis** The gentle twisting motion opens up the spinal canal, reducing compression on the spinal cord and nerves.	» **Sciatica** Stretching the hip flexors and strengthening the lower body can reduce sciatic nerve compression.

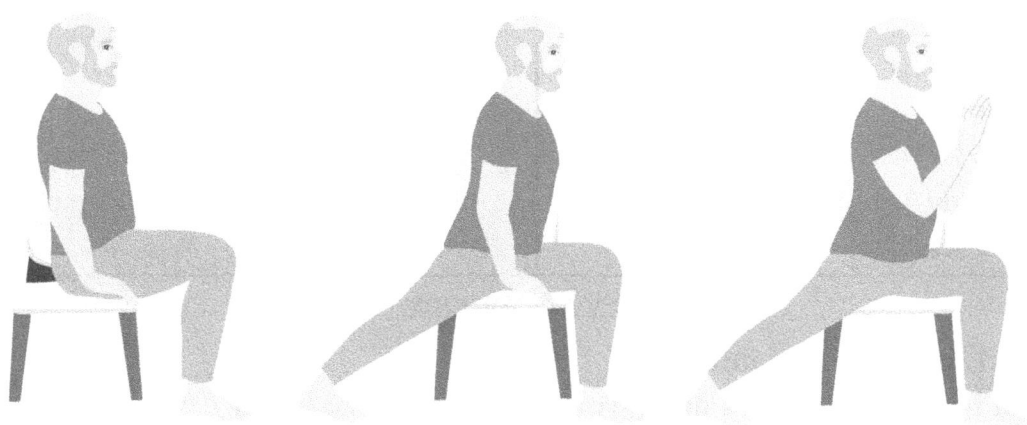

Steps:

1. Start by sitting upright towards the front edge of a stable chair, feet flat on the ground, turning your legs and body to the left side.

2. Extend one leg back, resting the foot on the ground, mimicking the stance of a traditional Warrior I but in a seated position. Ensure your front knee is directly over your ankle, forming a 90-degree angle.

3. Inhale and lace your hands in a prayer position at your heart center, engaging your core for stability. Draw your shoulders down away from your ears, engaging the core to support your spine.

4. Ensure your hips are facing forward, aligning your torso over your hips.

5. Hold the pose for several deep breaths, focusing on the stretch across your chest, shoulders, and the hip flexor of your extended leg.

6. To exit the pose, lower your arms and bring your extended leg back to the starting position.

7. Repeat on the opposite side to ensure balance in the stretch and strengthening of your body.

Chair Spinal Twist

<table>
<tr><td colspan="2" align="center">Helps with:</td></tr>
<tr>
<td>

» **Osteoarthritis**

This twist improves spinal flexibility and reduces stiffness in the vertebrae.

» **Spinal Stenosis**

The gentle twist opens the spinal canal, relieving pressure on the spinal cord and nerves.

</td>
<td>

» **Degenerative Disc Disease**

Twisting the spine helps maintain disc health by promoting movement and reducing pressure.

» **Sciatica**

The stretch in the lower back and hips helps alleviate tension and pain associated with sciatica.

</td>
</tr>
<tr><td colspan="2" align="center">

Safety Precautions:

- Twist gently and avoid straining.
- Consult a healthcare professional if you have severe back issues.

</td></tr>
</table>

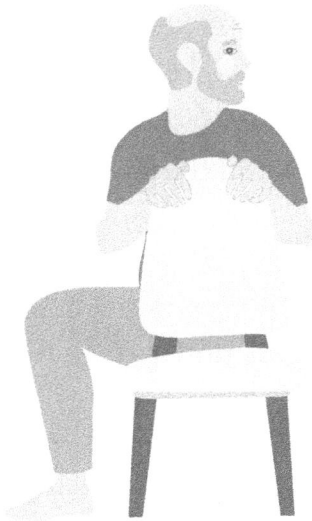

Steps:

1. Begin by sitting sideways on the chair, positioning yourself to face the left. This orientation prepares your body for the twist and ensures a full range of motion.

2. Grasp the back of the chair with both hands, establishing a firm grip that will aid in deepening the twist.

3. Take a deep inhalation to prepare your body. As you exhale, engage your core and twist your torso to the left, using your hands for gentle leverage. Look over your left shoulder to complete the twist, ensuring the movement extends throughout the spine.

4. Hold this position for a few breaths, allowing each exhalation to deepen the twist slightly, enhancing the stretch and its benefits on the spine and abdominal area.

5. To switch sides, gently release the twist and turn to face the right side of the chair. Repeat the twisting motion on this side to ensure a balanced, symmetrical stretch.

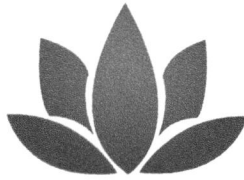

CHAPTER 3
CHAIR YOGA FOR JOINT AND ARTHRITIS PAIN

Joint and arthritis pain can really put a damper on your day, making even the simplest activities feel like a chore. Whether it's your knees, hands, hips, spine, shoulders, or feet, this pain can be relentless. But don't worry, we've got a game plan. We're about to dive into some powerful chair yoga exercises specifically designed to tackle these issues head-on.

Chair yoga offers a gentle yet effective approach to managing arthritis pain. These exercises are tailored to help you move better, feel better, and live better. Forget the days when pain dictated your schedule. With these exercises, you'll find relief and reclaim your pain-free lifestyle. Let's dive in and make those joints feel young again!

Now, let's get into the nitty-gritty of why chair yoga is so effective for managing arthritis and joint pain. Understanding the science behind it will help you appreciate just how beneficial it can be for your body.

WHY CHAIR YOGA HELPS WITH ARTHRITIS AND JOINT PAIN

» **Osteoarthritis**: This degenerative joint disease results from wear and tear on your joints, leading to pain, stiffness, and reduced mobility. Chair yoga helps by focusing on three specific things:

- Increasing Flexibility: Gentle stretching improves the range of motion, reducing stiffness and making daily activities easier.
- Strengthening Muscles: Building muscle around affected joints provides better support and reduces the load on the joints.
- Enhancing Circulation: This is a big one, improved blood flow from yoga movements helps nourish the joints and remove inflammatory waste products.

» **Rheumatoid Arthritis**: This autoimmune disorder causes inflammation in the joints, leading to pain and swelling. Chair yoga helps by:
- Reducing Inflammation: Gentle movements and stretching can help reduce joint inflammation and pain.
- Improving Joint Function: Regular practice helps maintain joint function and reduces the progression of joint damage.
- Promoting Relaxation: Yoga reduces stress and anxiety, which can lower the body's inflammatory response.

» **Overall Joint Pain:** Whether due to arthritis or other conditions, joint pain can severely impact your quality of life. Chair yoga helps by:
- Enhancing Mobility: Regular movement keeps joints flexible and prevents stiffness.
- Building Strength: Strengthening the muscles around joints helps protect and stabilize them.
- Increasing Endorphins: Physical activity, including yoga, releases endorphins, which are natural pain relievers.

CHAIR YOGA POSES FOR JOINT AND ARTHRITIS PAIN

Seated Knee Extensions

Helps with:	
» **Osteoarthritis** Strengthens the muscles around the knee joint, reducing stress on the cartilage and improving joint stability. This can help alleviate pain and reduce further degeneration. » **Overall Joint Pain** Enhances muscle support around the knee, increasing circulation and reducing stiffness and pain.	» **Rheumatoid Arthritis** Improves muscle strength and joint function, which can help reduce inflammation and pain in the knee joints.

- Extend your knee gently.
- Avoid if you have severe knee pain.

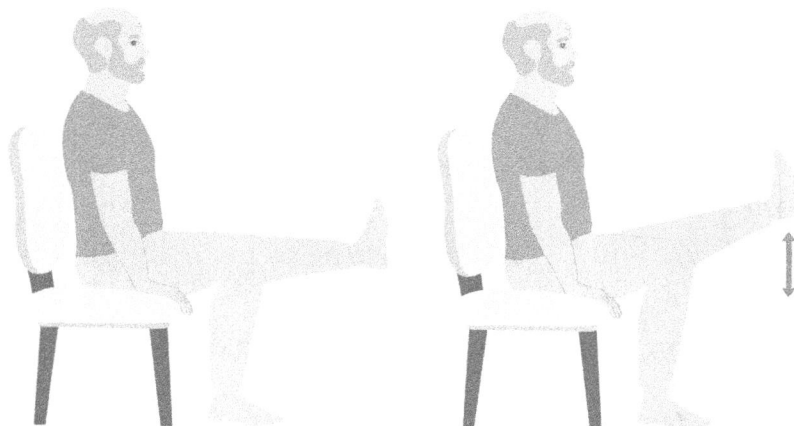

Steps:

1. Begin by sitting upright on a chair, ensuring your feet are firmly on the ground.

2. Extend one leg out in front of you, preparing for the lift. This action sets the stage for strengthening the muscles around your knee.

3. Slowly raise and lower the extended leg, maintaining a smooth and controlled movement. This precision helps in maximizing muscle engagement while protecting the knee joint.

4. Aim for 10-15 lifts, focusing on the quality of movement rather than speed. Each lift contributes to building strength in the thigh muscles and improving flexibility in the knee joint.

5. After completing the set, switch to the other leg to ensure balanced strengthening across both legs.

Seated Finger and Wrist Stretches

Helps with:	
» **Osteoarthritis** Improves flexibility and reduces stiffness in the fingers and wrists, helping to maintain mobility and reduce pain.	» **Rheumatoid Arthritis** Increases blood flow and reduces inflammation in the small joints of the hands, alleviating pain and preventing deformities.

» **Overall Joint Pain** Enhances flexibility and mobility in the fingers and wrists, reducing stiffness and discomfort.	

Safety Precautions:

- Perform the stretch gently to avoid overextension or strain on the wrists.
- If you experience any pain or discomfort during the stretch, ease up on the intensity or discontinue the stretch.
- Keep your movements slow and controlled, especially when extending your arms and pressing your palms forward.

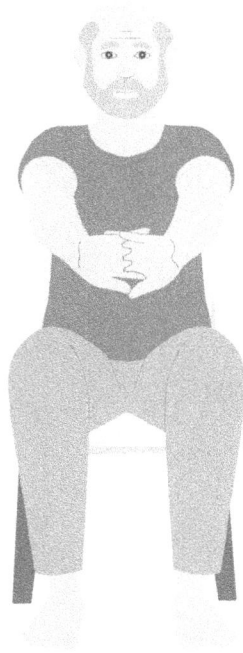

Steps:

1. Begin in a comfortable seated ensuring your spine is straight and shoulders are relaxed.

2. Gently interlace your fingers in front of you, ensuring a comfortable grip without squeezing too tightly.

3. With your fingers interlaced, flip your palms to face forward, away from your body. This action begins the process of engaging the wrists and forearms.

4. Carefully lift your arms to shoulder height, maintaining the interlaced fingers and forward-facing palms. Ensure your shoulders remain relaxed and down, away from your ears.

5. As you straighten your arms, press your palms forward, feeling a gentle stretch in the wrists and forearms. Ensure your arms are parallel to the floor, and you're pressing out as if against an invisible barrier.

6. Maintain this position for 5 deep breaths, focusing on the sensation of stretching and opening in the wrists and forearms. With each exhale, try to deepen the stretch slightly, without causing discomfort.

7. After holding for 5 breaths, gently release the interlace of your fingers and lower your arms back to your sides or lap. Shake out your hands and wrists gently if it feels comfortable.

Seated Hip Circles

Helps with:	
» **Osteoarthritis** Mobilizes the hip joints, increasing flexibility and reducing stiffness, which can alleviate pain and improve joint function. » **Overall Joint Pain** Enhances circulation and reduces stiffness in the hip joints, promoting better joint health and reducing pain.	» **Rheumatoid Arthritis** Helps maintain joint mobility and reduces inflammation in the hip joints, alleviating pain and improving overall hip function.
Safety Precautions:	
- Ensure the chair is stable. - Avoid this exercise if you have severe hip pain.	

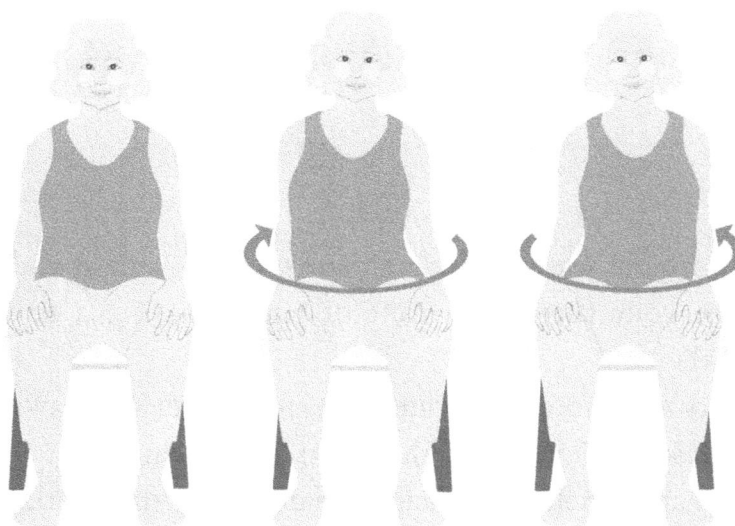

Steps:

1. Begin by sitting near the edge of a stable chair. Place your feet firmly on the floor, hip-width apart, establishing a strong foundation.

2. Rest your hands on your hips for added stability. This also helps in maintaining an upright posture throughout the exercise.

3. Initiate the movement by gently guiding your upper body in a circular motion to the right. Ensure the motion originates from the torso, engaging the muscles around the hip joint and lower back.

4. Continue the circular motion, moving your torso back, then to the left, and finally bringing them forward. This motion should be fluid and controlled, focusing on the range of motion that feels comfortable.

5. Complete five circles in this direction, then reverse the direction for another five circles. The reversal ensures balanced mobility and muscle engagement on both sides.

Seated Spinal Twist

Helps with:	
» **Osteoarthritis** Improves spinal flexibility and reduces stiffness in the vertebrae, which can alleviate pain and enhance joint function. » **Overall Joint Pain** Enhances flexibility and reduces tension in the spine, helping to alleviate overall joint discomfort.	» **Rheumatoid Arthritis** Reduces inflammation and pain by increasing blood flow and promoting better spinal alignment.
Safety Precautions:	
- Twist gently, avoiding any forceful movements. - If you have a spine condition, consult a healthcare professional first.	

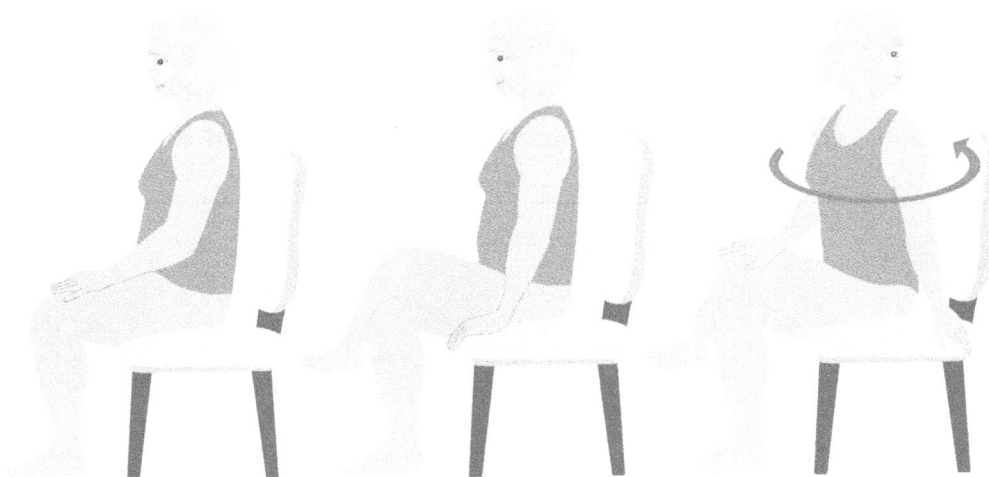

1. Begin by sitting upright on a stable chair, with your feet flat on the floor.

2. Cross your left leg over your right, placing your left foot beside your right knee. This setup prepares your body for a deeper twist and stretch.

3. Place your right hand on your left knee and your left hand behind you on the chair. These hand placements aid in supporting the twist and ensuring stability.

4. Inhale deeply to prepare your body. As you exhale, gently twist your torso to the left, aiming to look over your left shoulder. This movement initiates the twist from your lower back, extending up through your spine to your neck.

5. Hold the position for a few breaths, allowing the twist to deepen gently with each exhale. Focus on feeling the stretch throughout your spine.

6. After holding, slowly return to the center before repeating the exercise on the opposite side. This ensures balanced flexibility and mobility in both directions.

Shoulder Rolls

Helps with:	
» **Osteoarthritis** Improves circulation and reduces stiffness in the shoulder joints, which can alleviate pain and improve mobility. » **Overall Joint Pain** Enhances flexibility and range of motion in the shoulders, reducing stiffness and discomfort.	» **Rheumatoid Arthritis** Reduces inflammation and pain in the shoulder joints by increasing blood flow and promoting joint function.

Safety Precautions:

- Perform the movements slowly and gently to avoid any strain.
- Keep your spine straight and aligned to prevent slouching during the exercise.
- Breathe naturally, coordinating your breath with the movement for maximum relaxation.

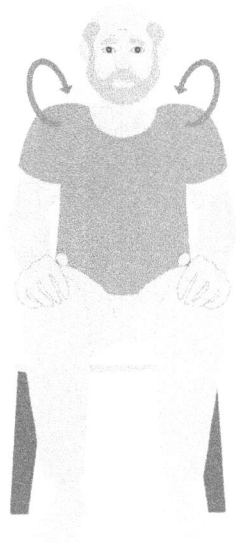

Steps:

1. Begin by sitting upright in a chair with your feet flat on the floor, hip-width apart, ensuring a stable and grounded posture. Place your hands on your thighs or let them hang by your sides.

2. Inhale deeply, and as you exhale, slowly lift your shoulders towards your ears, initiating the rolling motion.

3. Continue the movement by gently rolling your shoulders back, drawing your shoulder blades towards each other to open up the chest.

4. As you complete the backward roll, start to lower your shoulders down, creating a circular motion.

5. Once your shoulders are in their lowest position, begin the next roll by lifting them towards your ears again, then forward, up, back, and down, reversing the direction of the rolls.

6. Perform this circular motion slowly and smoothly for several repetitions, typically 5-10 times in each direction, focusing on the sensation of release and relaxation in your shoulder and neck area.

7. Pause for a moment after completing the rolls in both directions, taking a few deep breaths to settle into the relaxation and openness created by the exercise.

Seated Elbow Bends

Helps with:

» **Osteoarthritis**
Improves flexibility and reduces stiffness in the elbow joints, which can alleviate pain and enhance joint health.

» **Overall Joint Pain**
Enhances mobility and reduces stiffness in the elbows, promoting better joint function and reducing discomfort.

» **Rheumatoid Arthritis**
Increases blood flow and reduces inflammation in the elbow joints, alleviating pain and preventing joint damage.

Safety Precautions:

- Move in a controlled manner.
- If you have elbow or shoulder pain, proceed cautiously.

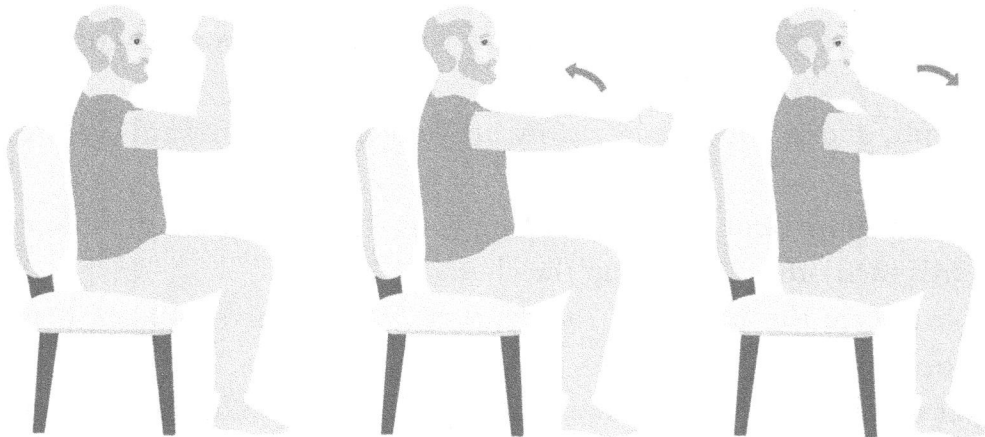

Steps:

1. Sit upright on a chair, ensuring stability and proper posture. This initial position is key for alignment and effectiveness of the exercise.
2. With arms extended forward and elbows bent at a 90-degree angle, you're positioned to begin the strengthening movement.
3. Smoothly extend your arms straight, then bend the elbows to bring your fists towards your shoulders. This motion engages the arm muscles in a controlled manner.
4. Repeat this bending and extending action 10-15 times, focusing on a fluid movement to maximize muscle engagement and joint mobility.
5. The controlled pace helps in focusing on muscle strength and joint flexibility, making each repetition effective.

Seated Calf Raises

Helps with:	
» **Osteoarthritis** Strengthens the calf muscles and improves circulation in the lower legs, which can reduce stiffness and pain in the ankle and foot joints. » **Overall Joint Pain** Increases circulation and reduces stiffness in the lower legs, alleviating pain and promoting overall joint health.	» **Rheumatoid Arthritis** Enhances muscle support around the ankle joints, reducing inflammation and pain, and promoting better joint health.

Safety Precautions:
-Move slowly and avoid jerky movements. - If you have ankle or calf injuries, proceed with caution.

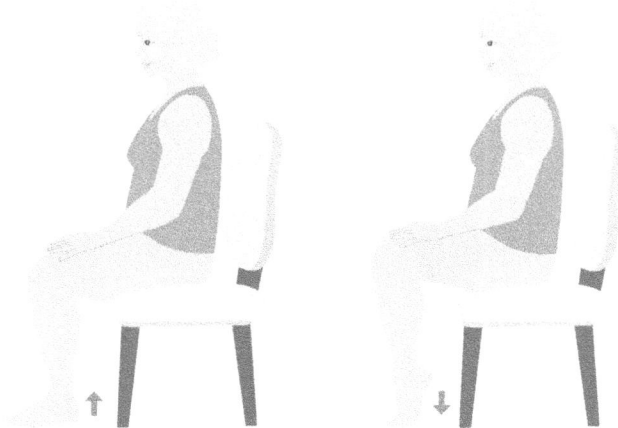

Steps:

1. Start by sitting upright in a chair with your feet flat on the floor. Ensure your posture is straight, supporting overall alignment and balance.

2. Gradually raise your heels off the floor, shifting your weight onto the balls of your feet. This movement engages the calf muscles, promoting strength and stability.

3. Hold this raised position for a few seconds. This pause is key to maximizing muscle engagement and enhancing stability in the ankles.

4. Gently lower your heels back to the floor, controlling the movement to ensure smooth and steady strengthening.

5. Repeat the calf raise 10-15 times. This repetition range is optimal for building strength and endurance in the calf muscles and ankles.

Alright, let's wrap it up. This chapter gave you the tools to fight back against joint and arthritis pain with targeted chair yoga exercises. By incorporating these gentle movements into your daily routine, you can reduce pain, enhance mobility, and improve your overall quality of life. Remember, consistency is key. Stick with it, and you'll start to see and feel the benefits.

Your journey to better joint health and less pain starts here. Don't let arthritis hold you back any longer. Embrace these exercises, stay committed, and watch how they transform your daily life. You've got this! Let's move forward together, stronger and more flexible than ever.

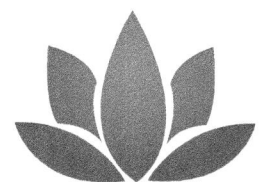

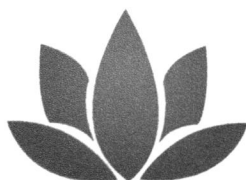

CHAPTER 4
CHAIR YOGA FOR UPPER BODY PAIN AND SHOULDER PAIN

Upper body and shoulder pain can be a real drag, especially when it stops you from enjoying your daily activities. Whether it's from cervical spondylosis, a herniated disc, muscle strain, rotator cuff injuries, frozen shoulder, or bursitis, these pains can make every move feel like a struggle. But don't worry—we're going to tackle these issues head-on with some gentle yet powerful chair yoga exercises designed specifically to reduce pain in your upper body, shoulder, and neck areas.

These exercises are designed to help you move more freely, allow you to reach higher shelves without discomfort, and enhance your overall well-being. Now, let's dive into the reasons why chair yoga is so effective for managing upper body and shoulder pain, especially for seniors. Understanding the science behind these movements will help you appreciate just how beneficial they can be for your body and mind.

WHY CHAIR YOGA HELPS WITH UPPER BODY AND SHOULDER PAIN

» **Cervical Spondylosis**: This condition, caused by wear and tear on the neck, can lead to chronic pain and stiffness. Chair yoga can help alleviate these symptoms by improving neck flexibility and strength. Gentle stretches increase blood flow to the cervical spine, reducing stiffness and discomfort, which is crucial for maintaining mobility and reducing pain as we age.

» **Herniated Disc**: When the discs in your spine press on nearby nerves, it can cause significant pain. Chair yoga helps by promoting spinal alignment and reducing nerve compression. Controlled movements and stretches relieve pressure on the discs and nerves, providing pain relief without the risk of overexertion.

» **Muscle Strain**: Overuse or injury can lead to muscle strain, making movements painful. Chair yoga exercises gently stretch and strengthen the affected muscles, promoting healing and reducing pain. This is particularly beneficial for seniors who need low-impact options to stay active and pain-free.

» **Rotator Cuff Injuries**: These injuries can cause shoulder pain and limit mobility. Chair yoga helps by strengthening the surrounding muscles and improving joint flexibility, which can alleviate pain and restore function, helping you maintain independence in daily activities.

» **Frozen Shoulder**: This condition restricts shoulder movement and causes pain. Chair yoga exercises gently stretch the shoulder joint, increasing range of motion and reducing stiffness over time, allowing you to regain mobility and perform everyday tasks more easily.

» **Bursitis**: Inflammation of the bursae, the fluid-filled sacs that cushion your joints, can be incredibly painful. Chair yoga helps by gently moving the affected joints, reducing inflammation and easing pain, making it easier to stay active and enjoy your favorite activities.

CHAIR YOGA POSES FOR UPPER BODY AND SHOULDER PAIN

Seated Neck Roll & Stretch

Helps with:	
» **Cervical Spondylosis** This exercise gently stretches the neck muscles, improving flexibility and reducing stiffness in the cervical spine. It helps increase circulation to the area, alleviating pain and reducing the risk of nerve compression.	» **Muscle Strain** Gently stretches and relaxes the neck muscles, reducing tension and pain caused by muscle strain. It promotes healing by increasing blood flow to the affected area.

- Perform movements gently to avoid strain.
- If you experience dizziness, pause and return to a neutral position.

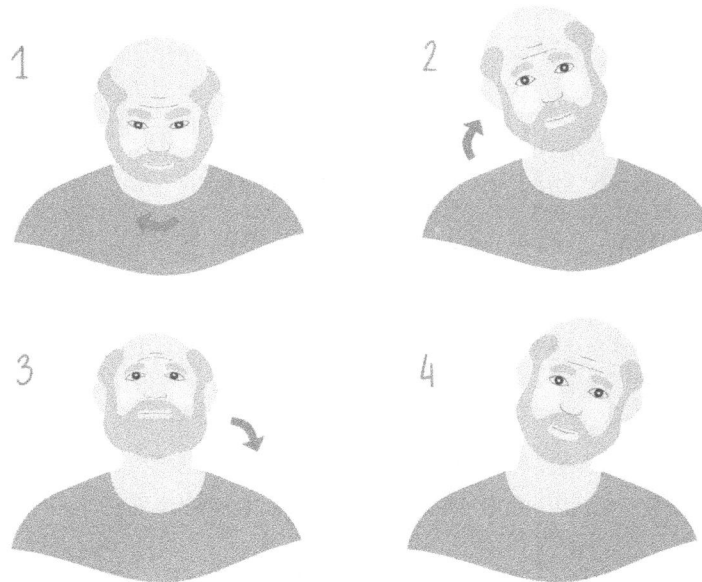

Steps:

1. Begin by sitting in a comfortable chair with your spine aligned and upright. This posture ensures a safe foundation for the exercise.

2. Slowly tilt your head forward, guiding your chin towards your chest. This initial movement starts the stretch and begins to release tension in the neck.

3. Gently roll your head to the right, aiming to bring your ear closer to your shoulder. This action stretches the side neck muscles, aiding in flexibility.

4. Continue the motion by rolling your head backward and then to the left, completing a smooth, circular movement. This sequence helps to evenly distribute the stretch across the neck muscles.

5. Perform 3-5 rolls in each direction, moving at a pace that feels comfortable and safe. Ensure each roll is performed gently to avoid any strain.

Seated Sun Salutation I

Helps with:	
» **Cervical Spondylosis** This series of movements increases overall spinal flexibility and improves posture, reducing strain on the cervical spine and alleviating symptoms.	» **Herniated Disc** Promotes gentle spinal extension and flexion, which can help alleviate pressure on the herniated disc and reduce pain.

» **Muscle Strain** Engages and stretches various muscle groups, improving overall muscle balance and reducing the likelihood of strain.	

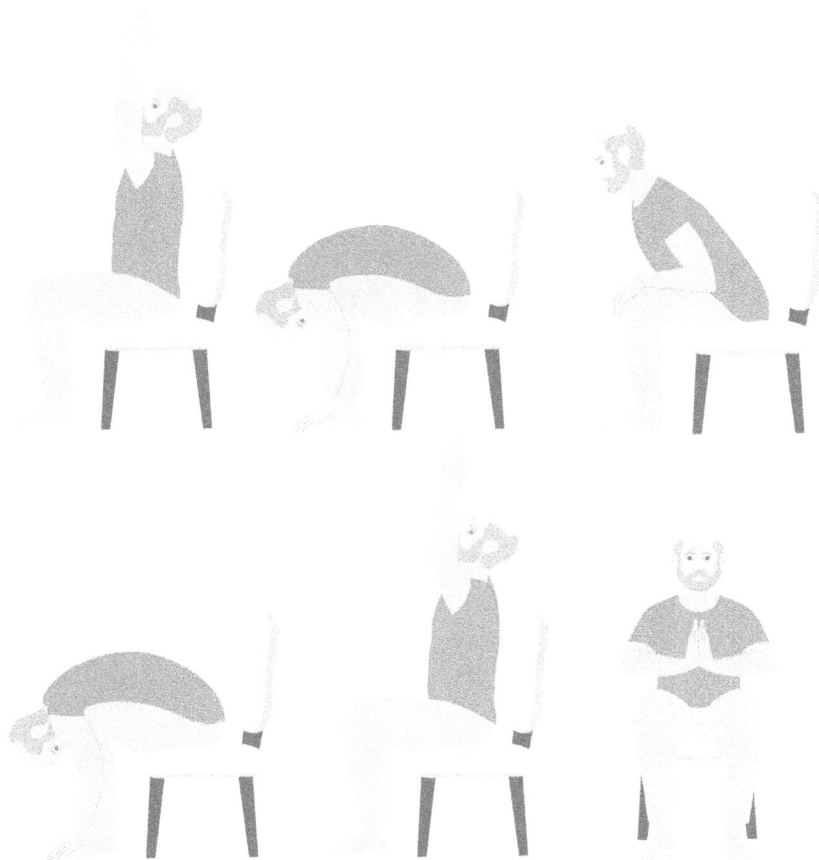

Steps:

1. Position yourself upright in a chair with your feet firmly planted on the ground, establishing a stable foundation.

2. Inhale deeply and raise your arms overhead, directing your gaze upwards, inviting energy and openness into your body.

3. Exhale and fold forward from the hips, extending your hands towards your feet. This forward bend encourages flexibility in the spine and legs.

4. Inhale and lift your torso halfway up, achieving a straight back. This movement helps to lengthen the spine and refresh the posture.

5. Exhale and fold forward again, deepening the stretch and promoting relaxation.

6. With another inhalation, rise up smoothly, stretching your arms overhead once more, embracing a full body stretch.

7. Exhale and bring your hands to your heart, centering your energy and focus as you conclude the sequence.

8. Repeat this sequence 3-5 times, flowing through each step with mindfulness and ease.

Seated Side-to-Side Lean

Helps with:	
» **Cervical Spondylosis** Improves lateral flexibility of the spine, reducing stiffness and alleviating pressure on the cervical vertebrae.	» **Muscle Strain** Gently stretches the muscles on the sides of the torso, reducing tension and pain from muscle strain.
» **Frozen Shoulder** Increases mobility in the shoulder joint, helping to alleviate stiffness and improve range of motion.	» **Bursitis** Reduces inflammation and pain by promoting gentle movement and increased blood flow to the affected areas.
Safety Precautions: - Lean gently to avoid strain. - Keep your buttocks firmly on the chair for stability.	

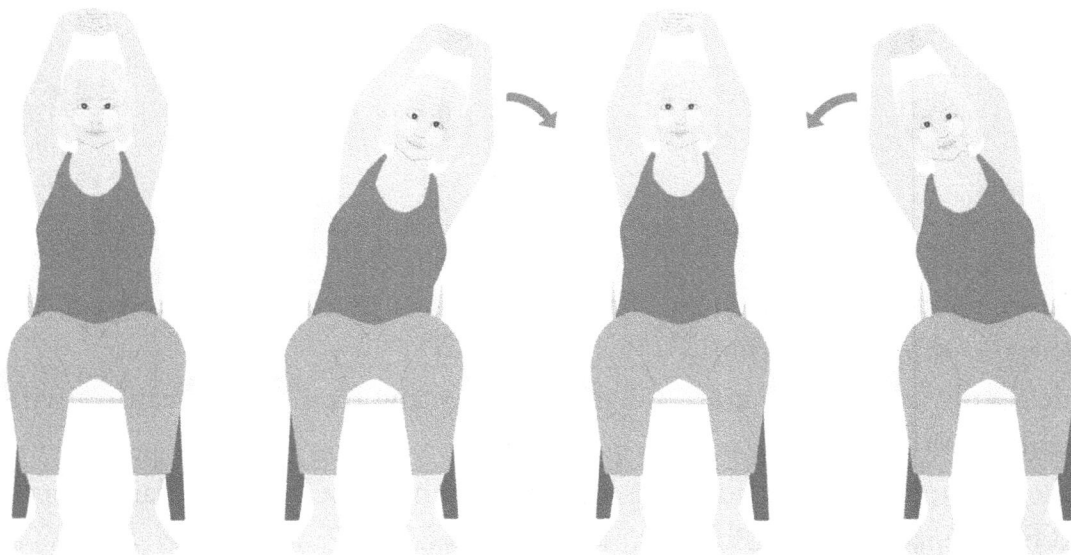

1. Start by sitting upright on a chair, with your feet planted firmly on the ground. This stable position ensures safety and effectiveness throughout the exercise.

2. Raise your arms overhead, interlocking your fingers with palms turned upward. This arm position helps maximize the stretch along the side body.

3. Take a deep breath in, and as you exhale, gently lean to the left, maintaining your extended arms. This movement stretches the right side of your torso, engaging the obliques and hips.

4. Inhale as you return to the center, preparing for the next stretch.

5. Exhale and lean to the right, stretching the left side of your body. This balanced approach ensures both sides of the torso are equally stretched and strengthened.

6. Continue this fluid, side-to-side motion for 5-10 repetitions, focusing on smooth, controlled movements. Each lean should be gentle to avoid any strain, with the buttocks remaining in contact with the chair for stability.

Seated Triangle Pose

Helps with:	
» **Cervical Spondylosis** Enhances spinal flexibility and improves posture, reducing pressure on the cervical vertebrae.	» **Muscle Strain** Stretches the muscles along the sides of the body, alleviating tension and reducing pain from strain.
» **Rotator Cuff Injuries** Engages and strengthens the shoulder muscles, promoting healing and reducing pain.	» **Frozen Shoulder** Increases shoulder mobility and flexibility, helping to reduce stiffness and improve range of motion.
Safety Precautions: - Use the chair for support and move into the twist slowly. - Avoid if you have severe balance or lower back issues.	

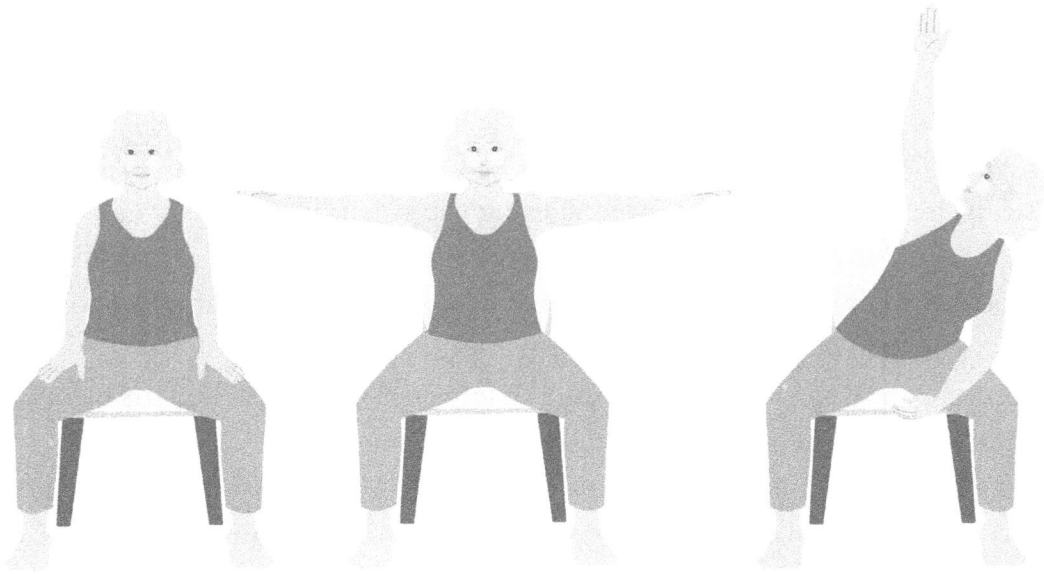

Steps:

1. Begin by sitting on your chair, opening your knees as wide as it feels comfortable, ensuring a stable and grounded posture. Make sure your ankles are directly aligned under your knees, with your toes pointing in the same direction as your knees to maintain alignment and stability.

2. Inhale and extend your arms to a T position at shoulder height, preparing your body for the side stretch.

3. Push your hips slightly to the right side, and as you exhale, lean towards your left thigh, keeping your back straight and elongated to maximize the stretch along your right side.

4. Rest your left forearm gently on your left thigh for support, and extend your right arm upwards, reaching towards the sky. This position creates a dynamic stretch along the entire right side of your body, from your hips to your fingertips.

5. Turn your gaze upwards towards your right hand, encouraging a slight twist in your upper spine and deepening the stretch.

6. Hold the pose for a few breaths, focusing on the sensation of stretching and opening through your right side, maintaining a long and straight spine.

7. To exit the pose, inhale and gently bring your torso back to the center, arms extended to the sides at shoulder height.

8. Repeat the stretch on the opposite side, pushing your hips to the left and leaning towards your right thigh, to ensure a balanced stretch on both sides of your body.

Chair Upper Body Twists with Arms Extended

Helps with:	
» **Cervical Spondylosis** Improves spinal flexibility and reduces stiffness in the cervical spine, alleviating symptoms.	» **Herniated Disc** Gentle twisting helps alleviate pressure on the herniated disc, reducing pain and promoting spinal health.
» **Muscle Strain** Engages and stretches the muscles of the upper body, reducing tension and pain from muscle strain.	» **Rotator Cuff Injuries** Strengthens and stretches the shoulder muscles, promoting healing and reducing discomfort.

Safety Precautions:

- Twist gently to avoid straining the spine.
- Keep movements controlled and avoid overextending the arms.

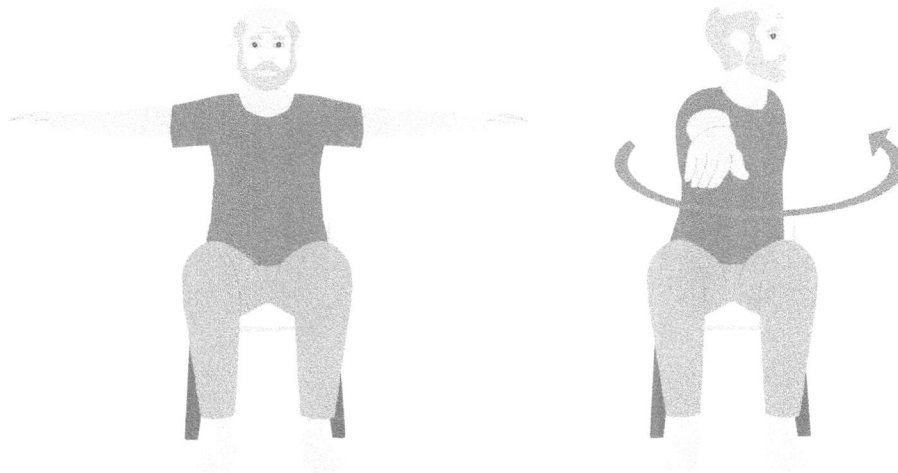

Steps:

1. Begin by sitting upright on a chair with your feet flat on the ground, establishing a stable base.

2. Extend your arms to the sides at shoulder height, creating a T-shape with your body. This position prepares your upper body for the twisting motion.

3. Gently twist your upper body to the left, ensuring your arms remain extended. This movement engages your core and stretches the spine, promoting flexibility.

4. Slowly return to the center before twisting to the right. This alternating pattern ensures an even stretch and strengthening across your body.

5. Continue this sequence for 10-15 repetitions on each side, focusing on controlled movements to maximize benefits and minimize the risk of injury.

Seated Star Pose

Helps with:	
» **Muscle Strain** Engages and stretches multiple muscle groups, reducing tension and pain from strain.	» **Rotator Cuff Injuries** Strengthens and stretches the shoulder muscles, promoting healing and improving range of motion.
» **Frozen Shoulder** Increases mobility and flexibility in the shoulder joint, helping to reduce stiffness and improve movement.	» **Bursitis** Promotes gentle movement and increased circulation, reducing inflammation and pain in affected joints.

Safety Precautions:

- Extend your arms and legs to a comfortable degree.

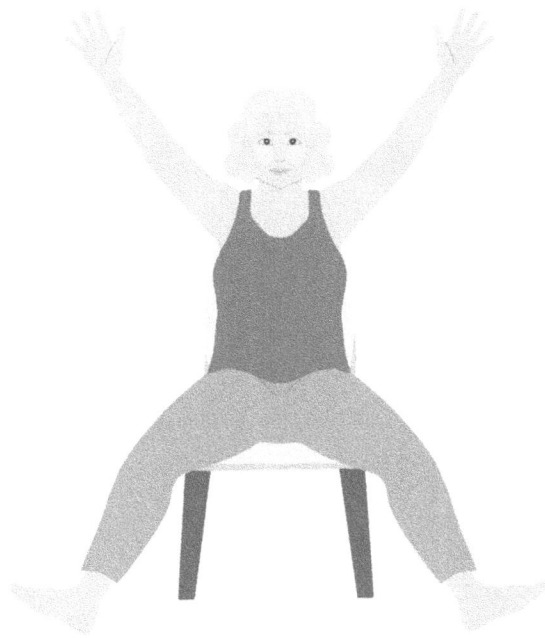

Steps:

1. Begin by sitting upright in a chair, ensuring your feet are planted flat on the floor for stability.

2. Gently extend your arms and legs outward from your body to form a star shape. This act of extension encourages the opening of the chest and the stretching of the shoulders.

3. Reach through your fingertips and stretch your toes away from the center of your body, intensifying the stretch across your chest and shoulders. This movement not only improves flexibility but also helps to strengthen the muscles involved.

4. Hold this expansive, star-like position for a few deep breaths, focusing on opening your chest with each inhalation and maintaining a strong, extended posture throughout the duration.

5. Gradually relax back to a neutral position, allowing your arms and legs to return to their starting positions.

Seated Locust Pose Variation

Helps with:	
» **Herniated Disc** Strengthens the muscles supporting the spine, reducing pressure on the herniated disc and alleviating pain.	» **Muscle Strain** Engages and strengthens the back muscles, reducing tension and promoting healing from strain.
» **Rotator Cuff Injuries** Strengthens the shoulder muscles, promoting healing and improving range of motion.	» **Frozen Shoulder** Enhances shoulder mobility and flexibility, reducing stiffness and improving overall function.
Safety Precautions:	
- Move slowly and avoid overstraining your back. - Not recommended for those with severe back pain.	

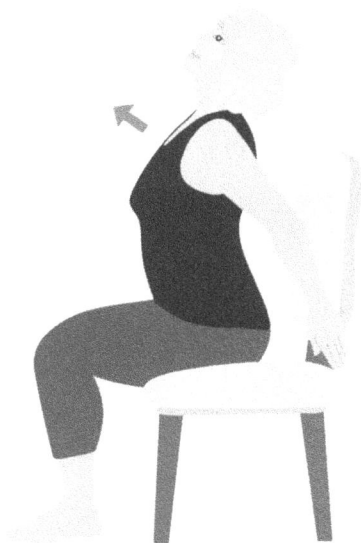

Steps:

1. Start by sitting at the edge of your chair, ensuring your feet are firmly planted on the floor. This position helps maintain balance and provides a solid foundation for the exercise.

2. Place your hands on your thighs or beside your hips, depending on what feels most comfortable and provides the best support for the upward movement.

3. As you inhale, gently arch your back, focusing on lifting your chest and shoulders upwards and backwards. This motion mimics the Locust Pose's back extension, activating the muscles in the lower back and spine.

4. For those who can and wish to deepen the stretch, extend your arms behind you, reaching away from your back. This optional step increases the intensity of the stretch, further engaging the back muscles and shoulders.

5. Hold this position for several deep breaths, concentrating on the stretching and strengthening sensations throughout your back.

10. To release the pose, exhale and slowly return to your starting position, allowing your back to relax before repeating if desired.

This chapter has equipped you with the right tools to tackle upper body and shoulder pain through targeted chair yoga exercises. By integrating these gentle movements into your daily routine, you'll find pain relief, improved mobility, and an overall better quality of life. Remember, consistency is crucial. Keep at it, and you'll begin to see and feel the positive changes.

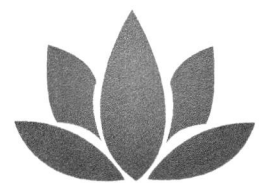

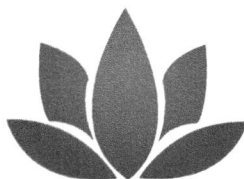

CHAPTER 5
CHAIR YOGA FOR COMBATING MUSCLE STIFFNESS AND PAIN

Muscle stiffness can be a real hurdle, especially when dealing with conditions like myofascial pain syndrome or fibromyalgia. These ailments often leave your muscles feeling tight, sore, and uncooperative. Fortunately, there's a way to combat this discomfort. We're going to tackle it head-on with some powerful chair yoga exercises designed specifically to alleviate muscle stiffness.

Chair yoga offers a safe, gentle way to stretch out those tight muscles and enhance your overall flexibility. These exercises are tailored to help you move more freely, reduce discomfort, and improve your quality of life. Imagine being able to play with your grandkids, work in your garden with ease, or take those morning walks without feeling stiff and sore.

Let's take a closer look at why chair yoga is so effective in relieving muscle stiffness. By understanding these benefits, you'll realize how much these exercises can improve both your physical and mental well-being.

WHY CHAIR YOGA HELPS WITH MUSCLE STIFFNESS

» **Myofascial Pain Syndrome**: This condition causes chronic pain in the connective tissues (fascia) that cover your muscles. Chair yoga can help alleviate this pain by gently stretching and relaxing the affected muscles, which can reduce tension and improve blood flow. Regular practice can help break up tight areas known as trigger points, providing much-needed relief.

» **Fibromyalgia**: This disorder is characterized by widespread musculoskeletal pain, often accompanied by fatigue, sleep, memory, and mood issues. Chair yoga helps by promoting relaxation and reducing muscle stiffness through gentle, controlled movements. The mind-body connection fostered by yoga can also help reduce the perception of pain and improve overall well-being.

CHAIR YOGA POSES FOR FOR COMBATING MUSCLE STIFFNESS AND PAIN

Seated Shoulder Shrugs

Helps with:	
» **Muscle Stiffness** This exercise helps to release tension in the shoulders and neck, improving circulation and reducing stiffness.	» **Myofascial Pain Syndrome** Shoulder shrugs can help relieve tightness in the shoulder muscles, which are common trigger points for myofascial pain.
» **Fibromyalgia** Gentle movements like shoulder shrugs can help increase blood flow and reduce overall muscle tension, which may alleviate some of the widespread pain and discomfort associated with fibromyalgia.	
Safety Precautions:	
- Move slowly and avoid overexerting the shoulder muscles.	

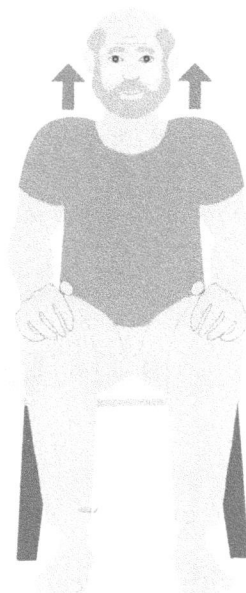

1. Sit upright in a chair with your feet firmly planted on the floor. This stable base supports proper posture and alignment throughout the exercise.

2. Inhale deeply, and with intention, lift your shoulders towards your ears. This upward movement should be controlled, engaging the muscles without straining them.

3. As you exhale, consciously release your shoulders back down. This downward motion encourages relaxation and the release of any built-up tension.

4. Repeat the shrugging motion 5-10 times, focusing on smooth, deliberate movements. Each shrug should contribute to a greater sense of ease in your shoulders and neck.

Seated Chest Opener

Helps with:	
» **Muscle Stiffness** This pose stretches the chest and shoulders, improving flexibility and reducing stiffness in the upper body.	» **Myofascial Pain Syndrome** Opening the chest helps release tension in the pectoral muscles, which can be trigger points for myofascial pain.
» **Fibromyalgia** By improving posture and reducing muscle tension, this pose can help alleviate some of the chronic pain and stiffness experienced by individuals with fibromyalgia.	
Safety Precautions: - Move slowly and avoid overexerting the shoulder muscles.	

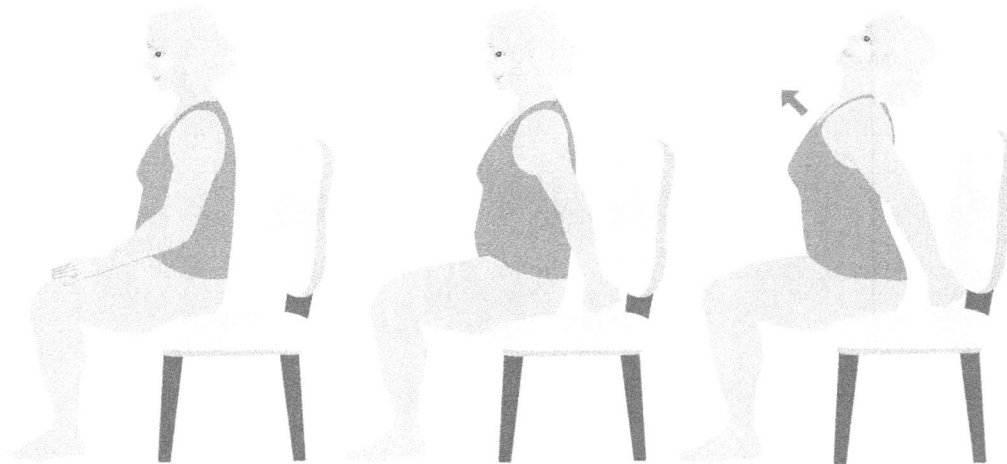

Steps:

1. Begin by sitting upright in a chair with your feet firmly planted on the floor. This stable position ensures proper alignment and support throughout the exercise.

2. Clasp your hands behind your back. This action prepares your upper body for the stretch and helps in engaging the correct muscles.

3. Inhale deeply, and as you exhale, gently pull your clasped hands downwards. Simultaneously, open your chest and lift your gaze slightly upwards. This movement stretches the chest and shoulders, encouraging a natural opening of the upper body.

4. Hold this position for several breaths, allowing the stretch to deepen with each exhale. The focus should be on maintaining a gentle stretch that opens the chest without straining the back.

5. Carefully release the stretch and relax. The controlled return to a relaxed state helps in maximizing the benefits of the stretch while ensuring safety.

Chair Lotus Pose Variation

Helps with:	
» **Muscle Stiffness** This pose gently stretches the hips and thighs, improving flexibility and reducing stiffness in the lower body.	» **Myofascial Pain Syndrome** Helps to release tension in the hip and thigh muscles, which are common areas affected by myofascial pain.
» **Fibromyalgia** By promoting relaxation and stretching key muscle groups, this pose can help reduce the widespread muscle pain and stiffness associated with fibromyalgia.	
Safety Precautions:	
- Ensure movements into and out of the pose are gentle to avoid straining the hips, knees, or ankles. - Listen to your body and adjust the pose as necessary to avoid discomfort.	

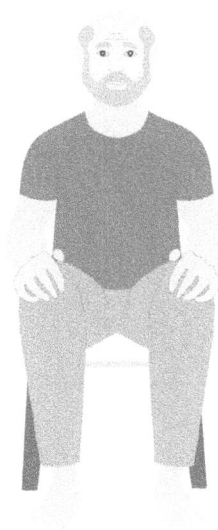

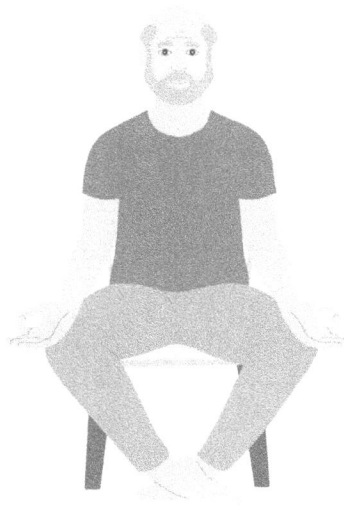

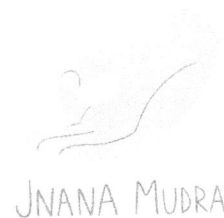

JNANA MUDRA

1. Start seated comfortably towards the front of a stable chair, keeping your feet flat on the floor to start. Ensure your spine is erect, promoting an aligned posture.

2. Gently cross your ankles in front of you, allowing them to stay close to the floor. This position should create a mild, comfortable stretch in the hips without the intensity of the full Lotus position.

3. Bring the backs of your hands to rest on your knees. Form Jnana Mudra by touching each thumb to its respective index finger, creating a circle, while keeping the rest of your fingers extended. This mudra is known for promoting wisdom and concentration.

4. With your ankles crossed and hands in Jnana Mudra, sit tall and breathe deeply. Allow your shoulders to relax away from your ears, and close your eyes if comfortable to enhance the meditative aspect of the pose.

5. Stay in this pose for several deep breaths, focusing on the sensation of relaxation and openness in your hips and lower back. Use this time to cultivate a sense of inner peace and calm.

6. To release, gently uncross your ankles and place your feet flat on the floor. Relax your hands and take a moment to notice any sensations in your body.

Seated Knee-to-Chest Lifts with Side Stretch

Helps with:	
» **Muscle Stiffness** This exercise helps to stretch and mobilize the lower back and hip muscles, reducing stiffness and improving flexibility.	» **Myofascial Pain Syndrome** Knee-to-chest lifts can help release tension in the lower back and hip muscles, which are common trigger points for myofascial pain.
» **Fibromyalgia** The gentle movement and stretching involved in this exercise can help alleviate muscle tension and improve overall mobility, reducing the impact of fibromyalgia on daily activities.	
Safety Precautions:	
- Perform knee lifts gently to avoid hip strain. - Ensure the chair is stable to prevent slipping or tipping.	

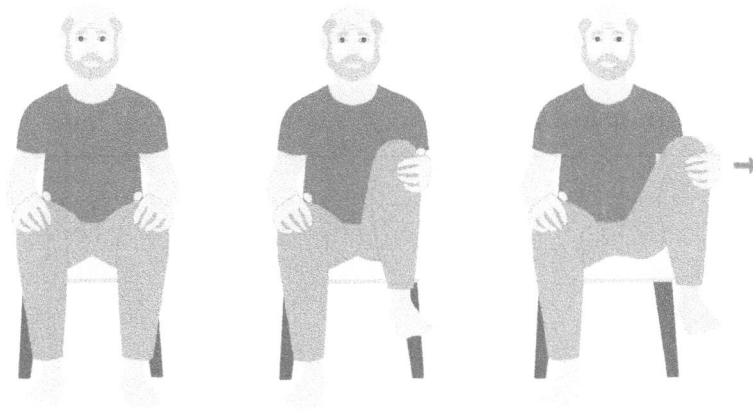

<u>Steps:</u>

1. Begin by sitting upright in a chair with your feet flat on the floor, creating a stable base for the exercise.

2. Gently lift one knee towards your chest, using your hands for support. If comfortable, gently pull the knee closer to your body to enhance the stretch in the hip and engage the core muscles further.

3. Hold this knee-to-chest position for a few seconds, actively engaging your abdominal muscles to deepen the core workout.

4. For the bonus side stretch, slowly hug the knee out to the side of your body, aiming to keep your back straight and engaging your side muscles for an added stretch. This movement not only aids in hip mobility but also stretches the side abdominal muscles, enhancing flexibility.

5. Carefully return the leg to the starting position, maintaining control and stability.

6. Repeat the knee-to-chest lift and side stretch with the opposite leg, ensuring an even workout on both sides. Alternate legs for 10-15 repetitions per leg to achieve a balanced strengthening and stretching session.

Seated Warrior II

<u>Helps with:</u>	
» **Muscle Stiffness** This pose strengthens and stretches the legs and arms, improving overall muscle flexibility and reducing stiffness.	» **Myofascial Pain Syndrome** Helps to relieve tension in the legs and upper body, which can be areas affected by myofascial pain.
» **Fibromyalgia** By promoting muscle engagement and flexibility, this pose can help alleviate some of the chronic muscle pain and stiffness associated with fibromyalgia.	

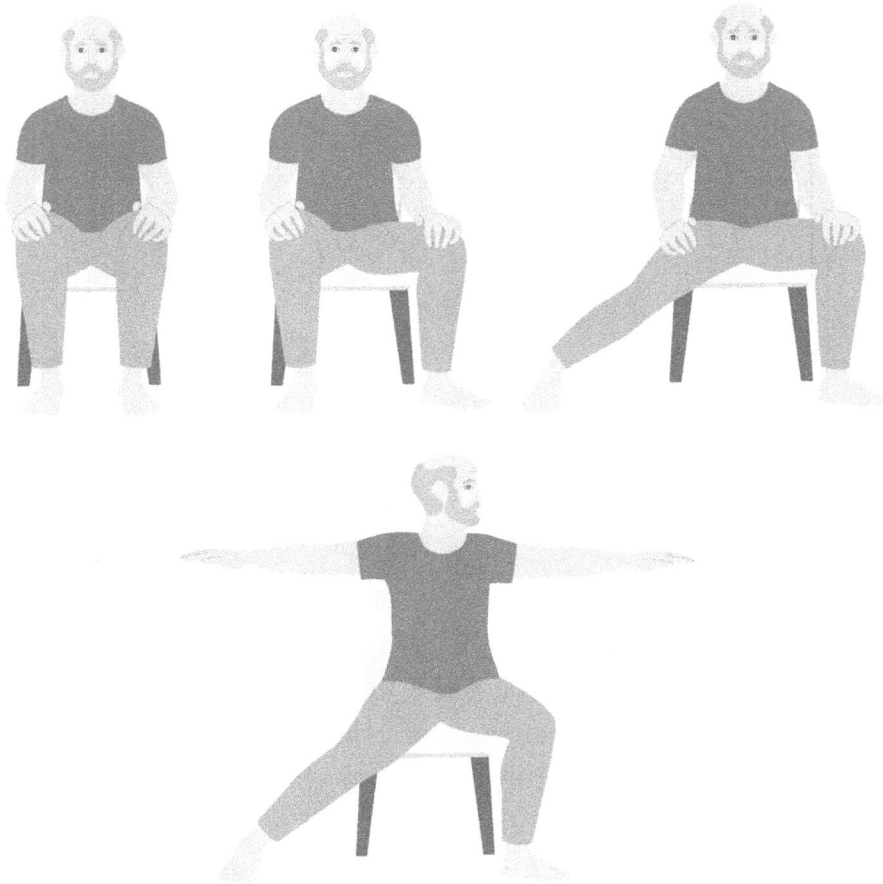

Steps:

1. Begin by sitting on the edge of a chair, ensuring your spine is erect and your hands gently rest on your knees. Your feet should be flat on the floor, spaced apart at shoulder width for a stable foundation.

2. Open your left leg to the side, creating a 90-degree angle at the knee, with your foot firmly planted and toes pointing to the left. This movement begins the process of opening up the hips and strengthening the thigh muscles.

3. Extend your right leg back, straightening the knee, and place your foot flat on the ground with your toes pointing forward. This position stretches the hip flexors and calves, contributing to the overall strengthening of the lower body.

4. Elevate your arms to shoulder height, reaching them outward to the sides in a powerful stance. This not only strengthens the arms and shoulders but also helps in maintaining balance.

5. Turn your head to gaze towards your left hand, aligning your focus with your body's direction. Hold this posture for three to four deep breaths, feeling the strength and stability in your pose.

6. To release, gently turn your head back to the center, lower your arms, and bring your legs back to the initial position. This careful, controlled movement ensures a safe and effective practice.

7. Repeat the pose on the other side: Shift your right leg to the side this time, creating a 90-degree angle at the knee, and extend your left leg back. Turn your head to gaze towards your right hand. Hold for three to four breaths before returning to the starting position.

Seated Forward Bend

Helps with:	
» **Muscle Stiffness** This pose stretches the entire back of the body, including the spine, hamstrings, and calves, reducing stiffness and improving flexibility.	» **Myofascial Pain Syndrome** Forward bending helps to release tension in the back and leg muscles, which are common trigger points for myofascial pain.
» **Fibromyalgia** The gentle stretch and relaxation of this pose can help reduce the widespread muscle pain and stiffness experienced by individuals with fibromyalgia.	
Safety Precautions:	
- Bend from your hips, not your waist. - Avoid if you have severe lower back issues.	

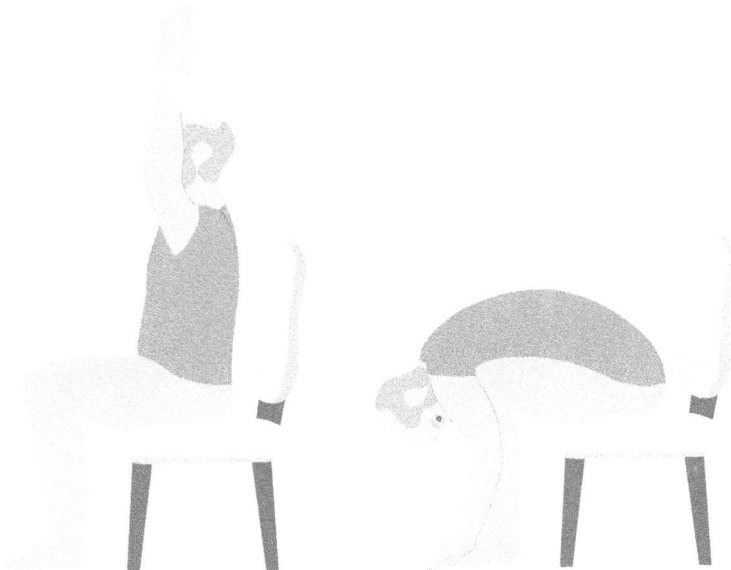

1. Start by sitting upright on a secure chair. Keep your feet planted on the floor, ensuring they are parallel and hip-width apart for stability.

2. Inhale deeply and raise your arms overhead, bringing a gentle stretch to your upper body. This upward movement also aids in elongating the spine.

3. As you exhale, gradually hinge forward from your hips, not the waist. This distinction is crucial for targeting the right muscles and ensuring safety.

4. Extend your hands towards your feet or shins, depending on your comfort and flexibility. The key is to stretch without straining.

5. Hold this forward bend for a few deep breaths, allowing the stretch to penetrate your spine and lower back. Focus on the sensation of release in your back with each exhale.

6. To conclude, slowly rise back to the sitting position, using your hands for support if necessary.

Seated Chair Pigeon Pose

Helps with:	
» **Muscle Stiffness** This pose targets the hips and glutes, stretching and reducing stiffness in these muscle groups.	» **Myofascial Pain Syndrome** Pigeon pose helps release tension in the hip and gluteal muscles, which can be trigger points for myofascial pain.
» **Fibromyalgia** By stretching and relaxing the hips and lower back, this pose can help alleviate some of the chronic muscle pain and stiffness associated with fibromyalgia.	
Safety Precautions:	
- Be gentle to avoid stress on the knee. - Avoid if you have severe hip or knee issues.	

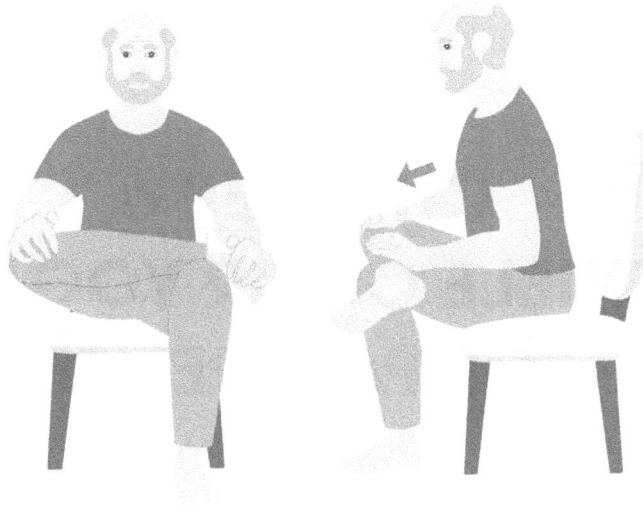

1. Start by sitting upright in a chair, ensuring your feet are grounded on the floor for a stable base.

2. Gently place your right ankle on your left thigh, just above the knee, creating a figure-four shape. This position initiates the stretch in the hips and glutes.

3. Allow your right knee to relax, avoiding any forceful pressing. For a deeper stretch, gently apply pressure to your right knee with your hand, increasing the stretch in the outer hip and thigh.

4. Slowly lean forward, bending at the hips while keeping your spine straight and tall until you feel a stretch in your lower back.

5. Hold this position for several breaths, focusing on deep, steady breathing to facilitate relaxation and deepen the stretch.

6. Carefully release your leg and switch to the other side, repeating the pose to ensure balanced flexibility and relief in both hips.

Alright, let's wrap this up. You've now got the tools you need to tackle muscle stiffness with targeted chair yoga exercises. By adding these gentle movements to your daily routine, you'll experience less stiffness, greater flexibility, and an improved quality of life. Stick with it consistently, and you'll start to notice and feel the positive changes.

Now on to the final chapter and creating your routine to bring it all together.

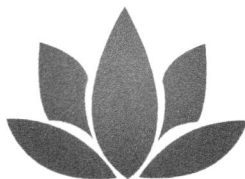

CHAPTER 6
YOUR FLEXIBLE CHAIR YOGA ROUTINE FOR PAIN RELIEF

To help you get started, here is a sample weekly routine plan. This plan is designed to be flexible, allowing you to easily adjust and change the exercises based on which areas are causing you the most pain.

Instructions:

1. **Begin each day with a breathing technique and some warm-up exercises.** This will help to center your mind and prepare your body for the chair yoga session.

2. **Follow the sequence of poses as outlined for each day.** Hold each pose for 30 - 45 seconds based on how you feel.

3. **Take a short pause of 15 seconds between each exercise or pose.** Use this time to breathe normally and prepare for the next pose.

4. **Remember to go at your own pace.** It's important to listen to your body and not push beyond comfort. If you experience any discomfort, modify the pose or skip it as needed.

5. **Begin with the goal of practicing these chair yoga workouts daily.** I know that you're busy, but I've found that this consistent approach helps students to establish a routine and maximize the benefits of the program.
   » However, it's important to listen to your body and be mindful of your energy levels and physical comfort.
   » If you find that daily practice is too demanding, or if you experience any discomfort, it's perfectly fine to adjust your schedule.
   » In such cases, aim to complete the workouts 4 to 5 times a week instead.
   » This adjustment ensures that you still maintain regular practice while giving your body adequate time to rest and recover.

I'm here to support you on your journey to a healthier, happier life. If you have any questions, concerns, or would like a few words of encouragement, please don't hesitate to reach out (jcharrisonbooks@gmail.com).

Here is an example of what doing some exercises from Part II - chapter 3 might look like.

WEEK 1 SAMPLE ROUTINE FOR PAIN RELIEF

Box Breathing (perform for 30-45s, page 22)

INHALE 4 SECONDS   HOLD 4 SECONDS   EXHALE 4 SECONDS   HOLD 4 SECONDS

Ankle and Wrist Rotations (30-45s, page 31)	Torso Twists (30-45s, page 30)	Shoulder Rolls (30-45s, page 111)

Seated Spinal Twist (30-45s, page 109)	Seated Calf Raises (30-45s, page 113)	Seated Elbow Bends (30-45s, page 112)

Remember to take a short pause of 15 seconds between each exercise or pose.

For week 2 feel free to try some of the other exercises from Chapter 3 or you can do exercises from a different chapter to target another pain point in your body.

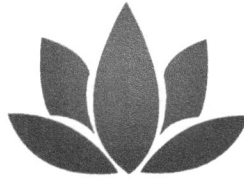

CONCLUSION

Let's take a moment to revisit the journey we've embarked on together. Throughout this book, we've delved into the powerful world of chair yoga, unveiling its transformative potential for pain management. We've explored how gentle, accessible movements can significantly reduce discomfort, enhance mobility, and improve overall quality of life. Chair yoga is a powerful tool in your arsenal, helping you combat pain while boosting your flexibility, strength, and mental well-being. Each chapter has equipped you with practical exercises and valuable insights to manage pain effectively, empowering you to take control of your health and live more comfortably.

Now, here's the real deal: consistency is key. Chair yoga isn't a quick fix; it's a lifestyle. The benefits you've started to experience—reduced pain, improved flexibility, better mood—are just the beginning. Stick with it. Make it a part of your daily routine just like brushing your teeth, the long-term rewards are immense. Picture yourself moving with ease, feeling more vibrant, and living a life with less pain. That's what awaits you if you stay committed.

Remember, every session builds on the last, creating a cumulative effect that will significantly enhance your overall well-being. And don't be discouraged by setbacks. Progress isn't always linear, but every effort you make is a step in the right direction.

Personal goals give you something to aim for and help maintain your focus. Start by setting achievable, short-term goals that lead up to your larger objectives. Use a journal or an app to track your daily practice, noting how you feel before and after each session, any improvements in your pain levels, and other positive changes you notice. This practice of self-reflection can be incredibly motivating. Celebrate each achievement—whether it's a week of consistent practice, a reduction in pain, or a new pose mastered. These small victories will keep you inspired and committed to your journey.

DEALING WITH PAIN MORE EFFECTIVELY

Managing pain is an ongoing process that requires a multi-faceted approach. Chair yoga is just one piece of the puzzle. Here are some strategies to enhance your pain management:

» **Mindfulness and Relaxation**: Incorporate mindfulness techniques into your daily routine. Practices such as deep breathing, meditation, or guided imagery can help calm your mind and reduce the perception of pain. By focusing on the present moment, you can shift your attention away from discomfort and create a more peaceful state of mind.

» **Regular Movement**: In addition to your chair yoga practice, ensure that you stay active throughout the day. Gentle movements, even if it's just a short walk or simple stretches, can keep your joints and muscles from stiffening up. Regular movement increases blood flow and releases endorphins, which act as natural painkillers.

» **Healthy Nutrition**: What you eat can significantly impact how you feel. A balanced diet rich in anti-inflammatory foods, such as fruits, vegetables, whole grains, and lean proteins, can help reduce pain and inflammation. Stay hydrated by drinking plenty of water, which aids in maintaining healthy joints and tissues.

» **Adequate Rest**: Your body needs time to repair and rejuvenate. Ensure you're getting enough sleep each night, as poor sleep can exacerbate pain. Establish a bedtime routine that promotes relaxation, such as reading a book, taking a warm bath, or practicing gentle yoga stretches.

» **Support Network**: Don't underestimate the power of community. Engage with others who are on a similar journey. Join support groups, participate in classes, or connect with friends and family who encourage and motivate you. Sharing your experiences and challenges can provide emotional support and practical advice.

» **Professional Help**: Sometimes, managing pain effectively requires professional assistance. Don't hesitate to seek help from healthcare providers such as physiotherapists, occupational therapists, or pain specialists. They can offer personalized strategies and treatments tailored to your specific needs.

EMBRACING A HOLISTIC APPROACH TO HEALTH AND AGING

Remember, pain management isn't just about the physical. It's about embracing a holistic approach to health. Your mental and emotional well-being are just as crucial. Chair yoga is a gateway to achieving this balance. It connects your body, mind, and spirit, fostering a sense of wholeness and well-being. Approach each session with an open heart and mind, and watch how it transforms not just your body, but your entire outlook on aging.

Embracing a holistic approach means recognizing that your body, mind, and emotions are interconnected. When you engage in chair yoga, you're not just moving your body; you're also calming your mind and lifting your spirit. This integrated approach helps manage pain more effectively by addressing its root causes. Alongside your physical practice, incorporate other healthy habits like balanced nutrition, adequate hydration, and positive social interactions. Use relaxation techniques, meditation, or breathing exercises to support your mental and emotional health. By nurturing all aspects of your well-being, you'll find a greater sense of balance and vitality as you age gracefully.

You've got this. Your journey to a pain-free, vibrant life is just beginning. Embrace it fully, and keep moving forward with strength and determination.

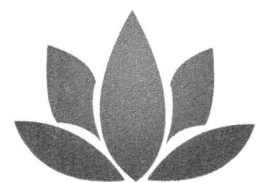

PART III
CHAIR YOGA
FOR STRENGTH

For Seniors To Lose Weight, Improve Mobility, Reduce Pain, Boost Bone Density & Gain Independence With Simple Seated Workouts in Just 10 Minutes a Day!

J.C. Harrison
Gran Publications

INTRODUCTION

Remember the thrill of a day spent in the garden, feeling the sun on your back as you planted flowers? Or the joy of chasing your grandkids around the park, their laughter ringing in your ears? Those moments of pure energy and vitality are priceless. But if the thought of kneeling to plant a flower or running after your grandkids feels overwhelming now, don't worry. You're not alone, and there's a way to get that strength back.

My name is JC Harrison, and I've dedicated my life to helping seniors reclaim their strength, mobility, and independence. Inspired by my own mother's journey to maintain her fitness and health as she grew older, I created a comprehensive chair yoga program tailored specifically for seniors. With years of experience in senior fitness and wellness, I help seniors become pain-free, increase their mobility, and regain their independence, all from the comfort of their chair!

My mission is simple: help as many moms, dads, grandpas, and grandmas play with their grandkids and live their golden years the way they always wanted. Through my books and our supportive online community, I aim to empower seniors to take control of their health and well-being. I believe that everyone, regardless of age or physical limitations, deserves to live a life full of vitality and happiness. My mission is to provide you with the tools and guidance needed to overcome mobility issues and rediscover the activities you love. Whether you're dealing with lack of strength, or stiffness, or simply looking for a way to stay active, I'm here to help you every step of the way

Chair yoga is your secret weapon for building strength without the high risk of injury from strenuous exercises. Think of it as your daily dose of power, right from the comfort of your own chair. When you integrate chair yoga into your routine, you'll start seeing some serious improvements. First off, core strength: we're talking about rock-solid stability that makes everyday tasks a breeze and slashes your risk of falls. Imagine standing up effortlessly or maintaining perfect posture while walking.

Upper body strength? We've got you covered. Strengthen those arms, shoulders, and chest, so lifting groceries or reaching for that top shelf becomes second nature. Now, let's talk lower body strength. Strong legs and hips are your foundation for mobility and balance. Chair yoga exercises target your thighs, calves, and glutes, helping you tackle stairs and longer walks with newfound confidence.

Balance and coordination are crucial, especially for preventing falls. Specific chair yoga poses will boost your stability, giving you the freedom to move without fear. Flexibility is your best friend here as it supports strength training by enhancing joint flexibility and muscle elasticity. Chair yoga stretches will keep your range of motion in check, making daily activities smoother.

Good posture is a game-changer. Strong muscles reduce strain and discomfort, and chair yoga promotes proper alignment, helping you sit and stand correctly. And let's not forget about circulation and cardiovascular health. Strength training benefits your heart by improving circulation. Chair yoga combines strength and flexibility exercises to boost your overall fitness.

By committing to chair yoga, you're taking control and prioritizing your health. You're choosing strength, stability, and a better quality of life. Don't take my word for it, just listen to what some of our community members have experienced:

Linda, a 78-year-old grandmother, shared in our Facebook group: *"Before discovering chair yoga, I was struggling with everyday tasks. Just getting out of my chair or reaching up to the top shelf felt like climbing a mountain. But since I started these exercises, everything's changed. I can lift my grandkids without any pain now, and I feel so much more independent and confident every day, thank you so much!"*

James, who is 72 and has been dealing with arthritis, posted: *"I was always on the lookout for an exercise that wouldn't make my arthritis worse. Chair yoga has been a lifesaver. I can move around with so much less discomfort. It's amazing how much stronger I feel."*

Betty, a 75-year-old passionate gardener, wrote: *"Falling was my biggest fear. My balance was awful. Your book has helped me so much. My stability and coordination have improved immensely. Now, I walk around my garden without any fear of tripping. It's given me my freedom back."*

Robert, who is 70 and recovering from hip surgery, shared: *"After my hip surgery, I thought I'd never get my strength back. JC you proved me wrong. These exercises helped me build muscle without straining myself. Now, I can climb stairs and walk longer distances, something I never thought possible a few months ago."*

These heartfelt stories from people just like you highlight the transformative power of chair yoga. Join us on this journey, and let's unlock your potential for a stronger, healthier, and more independent life.

This book is designed to guide you through a comprehensive journey of building strength through chair yoga, systematically covering all major muscle groups and aspects of physical fitness. Here's how the book is sectioned:

» **Core Strength**: We'll start with the foundation—your core. Strengthening your abdominal and back muscles is essential for overall stability and ease in daily tasks. This chapter will cover specific chair yoga exercises tailored for core strength, along with modifications for various fitness levels.

» **Upper Body Strength**: Next, we'll focus on building strength in your arms, shoulders, and chest. You'll learn specific poses and exercises targeting the upper body, with options to incorporate resistance bands or light weights for added benefits.

» **Lower Body Strength**: This chapter addresses the importance of strong legs and hips for mobility and balance. We'll explore chair yoga exercises that focus on your thighs, calves, and glutes, with techniques to safely increase resistance and challenge.

» **Balance and Coordination**: Maintaining good balance is crucial for preventing falls. You'll discover how muscle strength plays a role in stability and coordination through specific chair yoga poses designed to enhance these areas.

» **Flexibility and Mobility**: Flexibility is vital for supporting strength training and overall health. This section introduces stretches to improve joint flexibility and muscle elasticity, ensuring you maintain a good range of motion.

» **Posture and Alignment**: Good posture significantly impacts your overall well-being. We'll cover exercises that promote proper alignment and reduce strain, helping you sit and stand correctly throughout your daily activities.

» **Circulation and Cardiovascular Health**: Strength training also benefits your heart health. This chapter will highlight chair yoga techniques to improve circulation and combine strength with cardiovascular exercises for comprehensive fitness.

By structuring the book in this way, we ensure a well-rounded approach to building strength, focusing on different parts of the body and their specific needs. Each chapter builds upon the previous one, creating a holistic and effective chair yoga routine that empowers you to take charge of your health and well-being.

As you embark on this journey with chair yoga, remember that you are making a powerful choice to prioritize your health. By embracing chair yoga as a daily practice, you are taking proactive steps to alleviate discomfort and enhance your quality of life. Through dedication and consistency, you have the power to transform how you experience strength, balance, and mobility. This book is your guide to achieving a stronger, healthier, and more independent life. Together, let's unlock the benefits of chair yoga and embrace the potential for positive change within your body and mind.

CHAPTER 1
CHAIR YOGA FOR BUILDING STRENGTH

WHAT IS CHAIR YOGA WHY DOES IT WORK SO WELL AT BUILDING STRENGTH?

Chair yoga is your gateway to fitness, no matter your age or mobility level. Designed with seniors in mind, it adapts traditional yoga poses to be performed while seated or using a chair for support. This isn't about watering down yoga; it's about making it work for you. Chair yoga lets you reap all the benefits of yoga—flexibility, strength, balance—without the risk of injury or strain.

Imagine doing yoga without the worry of your knees, hips, or balance. That's the beauty of chair yoga. By using a chair, you can still experience the benefits of traditional yoga poses, but with a focus on what your body needs. It's about meeting you where you are and making yoga accessible for everyone.

Chair yoga includes a variety of poses and movements that target different muscle groups, increasing your strength, enhancing your flexibility, and improving your balance—all while seated or using the chair for support. Whether you're doing seated twists to engage your core, leg lifts to strengthen your lower body, or gentle stretches to improve flexibility, chair yoga offers a full-body workout that's both effective and gentle.

One of the main advantages of chair yoga is that it can be easily adapted to different fitness levels and physical abilities. This means that whether you're a seasoned yogi or completely new to working out, chair yoga can be tailored to suit your needs. Props like blocks and straps can be used to modify poses further, ensuring that each movement is within your comfort zone.

In essence, chair yoga is about accessibility. It opens up the world of yoga to seniors and anyone else who might find traditional yoga challenging. By making yoga practice more inclusive, chair yoga empowers seniors to take control of their health and well-being, improving their strength, flexibility, and overall quality of life.

IMPORTANCE OF CHAIR YOGA FOR SENIOR HEALTH

Chair yoga is your ticket to building strength, balance, flexibility, and better posture—essential for staying healthy as you age. Think about it: being able to lift your groceries without straining, get up from a chair with ease, or play with your grandkids without feeling wiped out. That's what chair yoga can do for you. It's all about making those everyday movements easier and more comfortable, reducing your risk of injury. Plus, better posture means less strain on your back and joints, leading to fewer aches and pains. By adding chair yoga to your routine, you're investing in a stronger, healthier you.

The mental perks of yoga are just as powerful. Regular chair yoga helps you stress less, focus better, and think more clearly. It's not just about moving your body; it's about boosting your confidence and mindset. Building strength through chair yoga gives you the assurance to handle daily challenges. The calming routine helps keep anxiety at bay and promotes a positive outlook. When you feel stronger and mentally sharper, you're ready to take on whatever comes your way with confidence.

Chair yoga classes are more than just exercise—they're a chance to connect with others. Whether you join a class in person or online, you'll find opportunities for social interaction that can reduce feelings of isolation. Our Facebook group takes this to the next level, giving you a platform to stay connected, share your progress, and stay motivated. The support and camaraderie from fellow participants can be incredibly uplifting, keeping you committed to your journey of building strength.

A regular yoga practice means a healthier, more active lifestyle. By making chair yoga a part of your daily routine, you're not just improving your quality of life—you're potentially increasing your lifespan. It's about staying strong both physically and mentally, so you can enjoy a longer, more vibrant life. Chair yoga keeps your body strong and flexible and your mind sharp and relaxed. This balanced approach to wellness means you're setting yourself up for a future where you remain active, engaged, and independent.

In a nutshell, chair yoga is more than just a workout; it's a holistic approach to building strength and enhancing your overall well-being. By focusing on both the physical and mental aspects of health, chair yoga helps you lead a balanced, fulfilling life. The physical benefits of improved strength and flexibility, the mental clarity and reduced stress, and the social connections you make along the way all contribute to a transformative practice that supports a healthier, stronger, and happier you.

THE 6 PILLARS OF STRENGTH

Building strength through chair yoga involves targeting several key areas: core, upper body, lower body, balance and coordination, flexibility and mobility, and posture and alignment. Each of these areas plays a crucial role in improving your overall health and making your daily life easier and more enjoyable.

» **Core Strength**

A strong core is the foundation of your overall stability and strength. When your core is strong, you'll find it easier to maintain your balance, reducing the risk of falls. Imagine being able to stand up from a chair without wobbling or feeling unsteady. A strong core supports every movement you make, enhancing your confidence and independence.

» **Upper Body Strength**

Building strength in your arms, shoulders, and chest is crucial for everyday tasks. Strong upper body muscles make it easier to lift groceries, reach for items on high shelves, and even hug your loved ones more comfortably. It's about making those daily activities less of a struggle and more of a breeze.

» **Lower Body Strength**

Strong legs and hips are vital for mobility and balance. Chair yoga exercises focus on the thighs, calves, and glutes, helping you walk longer distances and climb stairs with ease. With stronger lower body muscles, you'll feel more stable on your feet, reducing the fear of tripping or falling. Think about how empowering it would be to walk around your neighborhood or tackle a flight of stairs without hesitation.

» Balance and Coordination

Maintaining good balance is essential for preventing falls. Chair yoga poses designed to enhance stability and coordination, like the seated tree pose, help you move confidently without fear of stumbling. Improved balance means you can navigate your home and community with ease, avoiding accidents that could lead to injury. It's about moving through your day with a sense of assurance and grace.

» Flexibility and Mobility

Flexibility is a key component of overall health and supports strength training. Chair yoga stretches, such as seated forward bends and leg extensions, enhance joint flexibility and muscle elasticity, ensuring a full range of motion. Increased flexibility makes everyday movements smoother and less painful, from bending down to tie your shoes to reaching out for a handshake. Flexibility and mobility exercises ensure that your body can move freely and comfortably, reducing stiffness and improving your overall quality of life.

» Posture and Alignment

Strong muscles contribute to good posture, which in turn reduces strain and discomfort. Chair yoga exercises promote proper alignment, helping you maintain correct posture throughout your daily activities. Good posture alleviates back and neck pain and supports your overall well-being. Imagine sitting and standing with ease, feeling tall and aligned. Proper posture impacts how you present yourself to the world and how you feel internally, boosting both your physical and mental health.

By focusing on these key areas, chair yoga helps you build strength in a balanced and comprehensive way. This not only improves your physical health but also enhances your ability to perform daily tasks, boosts your confidence, and enriches your overall quality of life. Chair yoga isn't just about exercise; it's about empowering you to live your life to the fullest with strength, balance, and vitality.

WHAT CAUSES STRENGTH ISSUES AND HOW CAN CHAIR YOGA HELP?

Understanding why strength diminishes as we age is crucial to appreciating the value of chair yoga and the difference it can make in your life. Here's a deep dive into the factors contributing to muscle loss and how chair yoga can help combat these issues.

» Sarcopenia (Muscle Atrophy)

Sarcopenia, the natural loss of muscle mass and strength as we age, can make everyday activities increasingly difficult. From lifting a grocery bag to getting out of a chair, these tasks can become challenging. Chair yoga slows this process by continuously engaging and strengthening your muscles. Regular practice keeps your muscles active and helps maintain their mass, allowing you to perform daily tasks with more ease and confidence.

» Decreased Physical Activity

As we get older, it's common to become less physically active. This reduction in activity leads to muscle loss and decreased strength, creating a vicious cycle where it becomes even harder to stay active. Chair yoga provides a manageable way to stay engaged in physical activity, breaking this cycle. By incorporating gentle movements and strength-building exercises into your routine, chair yoga helps you stay active, preserving and even improving your muscle strength over time.

» Hormonal Changes

The decline in hormones like testosterone and growth hormone, which are crucial for muscle maintenance and growth, is another factor. Lower levels of these hormones contribute to muscle loss. Regular chair yoga can help maintain muscle health by promoting hormonal balance through gentle yet effective exercise. This helps offset the natural decline and supports muscle growth and maintenance.

» Nutritional Deficiencies

Adequate nutrition is vital for maintaining muscle health. Seniors are often more susceptible to nutritional deficiencies, especially in protein, which is essential for building and maintaining muscle. A balanced diet rich in protein and essential vitamins, combined with chair yoga, supports muscle growth and maintenance. The exercise routines help ensure that the nutrients you consume are effectively used by your body, promoting better overall muscle health.

» Chronic Conditions

Many chronic health conditions, such as arthritis, diabetes, and heart disease, can limit mobility and make exercising difficult, leading to muscle loss. Chair yoga offers a low-impact exercise option that can be tailored to accommodate these conditions. By keeping muscles engaged and active without overstraining them, chair yoga helps maintain strength and mobility even when dealing with chronic health issues.

» Medications

Certain medications can have side effects that contribute to muscle weakness or interfere with muscle function. Chair yoga helps mitigate these effects by keeping your muscles engaged and active. Regular movement and strength exercises counteract the weakening effects of medications, helping you maintain your muscle health.

» Inflammation

Chronic inflammation, common in seniors, can damage muscle tissue and hinder muscle growth. The gentle movements of chair yoga can reduce inflammation and support muscle growth. By incorporating anti-inflammatory exercises, chair yoga helps protect muscle tissue and promotes healing and growth.

» Reduced Nerve Function

As we age, nerve function can decline, leading to decreased signals from the brain to the muscles. This affects muscle contractions and strength. Chair yoga enhances neuromuscular coordination, improving muscle function. By regularly practicing chair yoga, you can help maintain and improve the communication between your brain and muscles, ensuring better muscle performance and strength.

» Changes in Body Composition

With age, body fat percentage tends to increase while muscle mass decreases. This shift in body composition contributes to a decline in overall strength and affects metabolism. Chair yoga helps maintain a healthy body composition by promoting muscle growth and reducing fat. The strength-building exercises ensure that your muscles stay active, helping you maintain a more balanced body composition.

» Psychological Factors

Fear of falling or pain can deter seniors from engaging in physical activity, leading to muscle loss and decreased strength. Chair yoga builds confidence through safe, manageable exercises, encouraging regular physical activity. By providing a secure environment to practice strength-building movements, chair yoga helps alleviate fears and motivates you to stay active.

» **Increased Independence and Daily Living**

Stronger muscles from chair yoga can transform your daily life, making everyday tasks easier and boosting your independence. When your muscles are strong, you can perform activities like getting dressed, climbing stairs, and carrying groceries with greater ease and confidence. This improvement in functional mobility means you rely less on others, which enhances your sense of autonomy. Imagine the freedom of being able to move around your home effortlessly or enjoy activities with your family without needing help. Chair yoga empowers you to reclaim your independence and live life on your terms.

» **Overall Health and Well-Being**

Chair yoga goes beyond just building strength; it significantly enhances your overall health and well-being. Regular practice improves bone density, helping to combat osteoporosis and reduce the risk of fractures. By engaging in chair yoga, you also boost your metabolism, which aids in weight management and supports cardiovascular health. These physical benefits are complemented by the mental health gains you'll experience. As you get stronger, your confidence grows, lifting your mood and enhancing your self-esteem. Chair yoga promotes a holistic sense of well-being, making you feel better both physically and mentally.

» **Sustainable Lifestyle**

One of the greatest benefits of chair yoga is its sustainability. It helps seniors stay active and engaged in physical activities, improving overall fitness and energy levels. Building strength now means supporting your physical capabilities for a longer time, leading to a more independent and fulfilling life as you age. Chair yoga is designed to be a gentle yet effective workout that you can maintain over the long term. By incorporating it into your daily routine, you ensure that you stay active and healthy, paving the way for a vibrant, energized lifestyle.

» **Reduced Fall Risk**

Falls are a major concern for seniors, but chair yoga can significantly reduce this risk by strengthening your legs and core, which improves balance and coordination. The targeted exercises in chair yoga help stabilize your muscles, making you less prone to falls. With better balance and stability, you can navigate your environment with confidence, avoiding accidents that could lead to serious injuries. Preventing falls is crucial for maintaining your health and independence, and chair yoga provides a practical and effective solution.

» Pain Management

Stronger muscles support your joints and improve your posture, which can reduce pain and stiffness associated with conditions like arthritis. Chair yoga offers a safe, low-impact way to manage and alleviate chronic pain. By regularly practicing these gentle exercises, you can decrease inflammation, increase joint mobility, and enhance your overall comfort. The movements in chair yoga are designed to stretch and strengthen muscles without causing strain, making it an ideal practice for pain management. This allows you to stay active and enjoy life with less discomfort.

In summary, chair yoga is a powerful tool for building strength and enhancing your overall quality of life. From increasing your independence and improving your health to creating a sustainable lifestyle and reducing fall risks, chair yoga addresses the unique challenges seniors face. By integrating chair yoga into your routine, you're making a commitment to a stronger, healthier, and more active life.

CHAPTER 2
CHAIR YOGA FOR CORE STRENGTH

Maintaining and enhancing core strength is crucial for overall stability, balance, and functional mobility, especially as we age. A robust core supports your spine, improves posture, and helps you perform everyday activities with ease and confidence. Weak core muscles can lead to poor balance, an increased risk of falls, and chronic lower back pain. Incorporating specific chair yoga exercises that target the core can strengthen these essential muscles safely and effectively.

Your core is not just about having firm abdominal muscles; it encompasses the entire area between your pelvis and ribcage, including your back and sides. These muscles are the foundation of your body, providing support and stability for almost every movement you make. A strong core is essential for maintaining balance, stability, and posture, which are critical for performing daily tasks efficiently and safely.

Think about the activities you do each day—standing up from a chair, bending down to tie your shoes, lifting groceries, or even reaching for something on a high shelf. All these movements engage your core muscles. Here's how your core plays a role in everyday tasks:

» **Standing Up and Sitting Down**: Your core muscles help you maintain balance and stability as you transition from sitting to standing and vice versa.

» **Bending and Lifting**: Whether you're picking up a laundry basket or reaching down to pet your dog, your core provides the necessary support to protect your back and prevent injury.

» **Reaching and Stretching**: Activities like reaching for items on a top shelf or stretching to open a window engage your core to keep you stable and prevent falls.

» **Walking and Balance**: A strong core improves your balance and coordination, making it easier to walk and navigate your surroundings safely.

By strengthening your core, you enhance your ability to perform these tasks with greater ease and confidence. This not only improves your quality of life but also reduces the risk of injury and promotes overall well-being.

CORE STRENGTHENING POSES

Now that you understand the importance of your core, let's move on to the exercises. Here are some chair yoga poses designed to target and strengthen your core muscles:

Seated Knee Lifts

Helps with:	
» **Muscle strengthening** This exercise targets the hip flexors and lower abdominal muscles, building strength in the core and legs.	» **Improved balance and coordination** Lifting the knees enhances coordination and stability in the lower body.
» **Improved circulation** The movement promotes blood flow to the lower extremities, improving overall circulation.	
Safety Precautions:	
- Lift the knee only as high as comfortable. - Avoid if you have acute hip pain.	

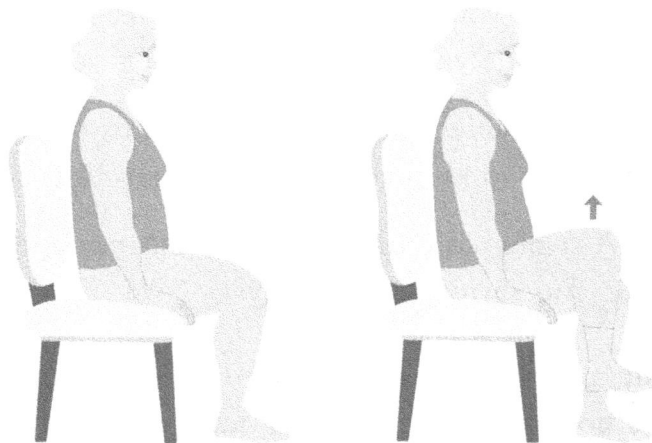

1. Begin by sitting upright on a stable chair, ensuring your feet are flat on the ground. This starting posture helps maintain balance and alignment during the exercise.

2. Place your hands on your thighs or the sides of the chair for additional stability. This support is crucial for maintaining proper form throughout the movement.

3. Slowly lift one knee towards your chest, keeping the movement controlled and the other foot flat on the floor. This action engages the thigh muscles and encourages hip mobility.

4. Hold the lifted position for a few seconds, focusing on engaging your core and thigh muscles. This hold increases muscle strength and stability.

5. Gently lower the leg back to the starting position, ensuring the movement is smooth and controlled.

6. Alternate legs, performing 10-15 lifts per leg. This repetition ensures balanced strength and flexibility in both hips and thighs.

Chair Cat-Cow Stretch

Helps with:	
» **Muscle strengthening** Engages the core muscles to transition between arching and rounding the spine, promoting abdominal and back muscle activation.	» **Improved balance and coordination** The rhythmic movement enhances coordination between the core and other muscle groups.
» **Enhanced joint flexibility** Increases flexibility in the spine, which aids in overall mobility and ease of movement.	» **Improved posture** Strengthening the core helps support proper spinal alignment, reducing the risk of slouching and poor posture.

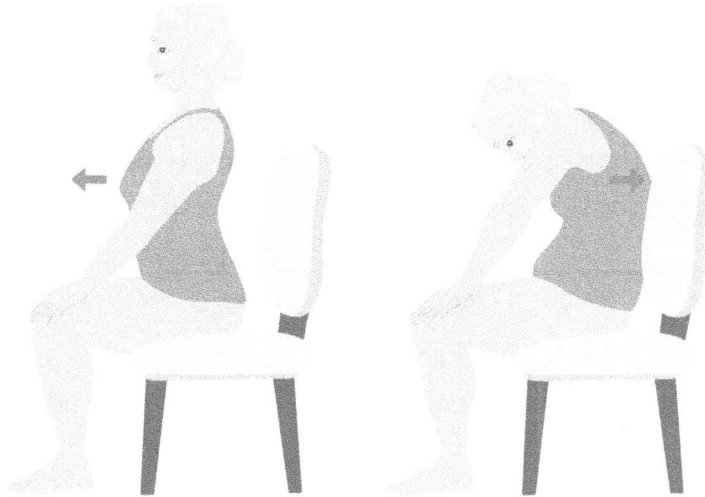

Steps:

1. Sit upright towards the front edge of a stable chair, placing your feet flat on the floor, hip-width apart. Place your hands on your knees or thighs for support.

2. Begin with the Cow pose: Inhale, arch your back, and tilt your pelvis back, sticking your buttocks out slightly. Lift your chest and chin upwards, gazing slightly forward or up, and pull your shoulders back. This position encourages a gentle arch in your lower back, opening the chest and stretching the front of your torso.

3. Transition to the Cat pose: Exhale, round your spine, and tilt your pelvis forward, tucking your tailbone under. Draw your chin towards your chest, gaze down at your navel, and push your mid-back towards the chair back. This movement stretches the back of your spine and releases tension in your neck and shoulders.

4. Continue to flow smoothly between the Cow and Cat poses, following the rhythm of your breath: Inhale as you move into Cow pose, and exhale as you transition into Cat pose.

5. Repeat this sequence for several breath cycles (typically 5-10), focusing on the sensation of movement along your spine and the relaxation of tension with each transition.

Chair Assisted Torso Twist

Helps with:	
» **Muscle strengthening** Actively engages the core muscles, particularly the obliques, to twist and stabilize the torso. » **Enhanced joint flexibility** Increases flexibility in the spine and helps maintain a full range of motion in the torso.	» **Improved balance and coordination** Twisting movements enhance coordination and stability by engaging the core and lower body. » **Improved posture** Strengthening the core muscles supports proper spinal alignment and helps maintain an upright posture.

<table>
<tr><td colspan="2" align="center">Safety Precautions:</td></tr>
<tr><td colspan="2">- Twist gently, avoiding any forceful movements.
- If you have a spine condition, consult a healthcare professional first.</td></tr>
</table>

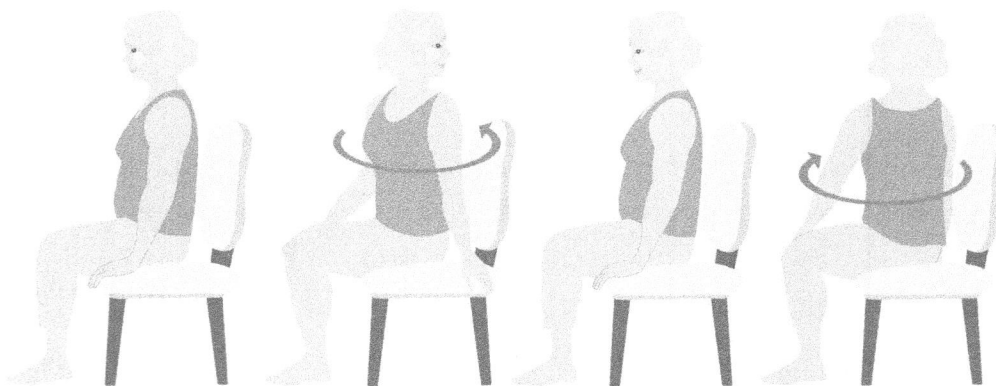

Steps:

1. Begin by sitting upright in a chair, ensuring your feet are flat on the ground. This position helps maintain balance and proper spinal alignment during the twist.

2. Place your right hand on your left knee and your left hand behind you on the chair. These hand placements provide stability and support for the twist.

3. Inhale deeply to prepare. As you exhale, gently twist your torso to the left. This movement should originate from the base of your spine, ensuring a gentle and effective stretch.

4. Hold the twist for a few breaths, allowing your body to relax into the position. This holding phase aids in deepening the stretch while supporting spinal health and digestion.

5. Slowly return to the center before repeating the exercise on the opposite side. This ensures balanced mobility and flexibility on both sides of the body.

Seated Side Bends with Weights

Helps with:	
» **Muscle strengthening** Engages the obliques and deep abdominal muscles, enhancing overall core strength.	» **Improved balance and coordination** The movement requires stabilization of the torso, improving balance and coordination.
» **Enhanced joint flexibility** Stretches the sides of the body, increasing flexibility in the spine and intercostal muscles.	» **Improved posture** Strengthening the side muscles supports proper spinal alignment, helping to counteract slouching and promoting a more upright and balanced posture.

<u>Safety Precautions:</u>

- Use light weights and move slowly to avoid strain.
- If you have shoulder or back issues, do this exercise without weights.

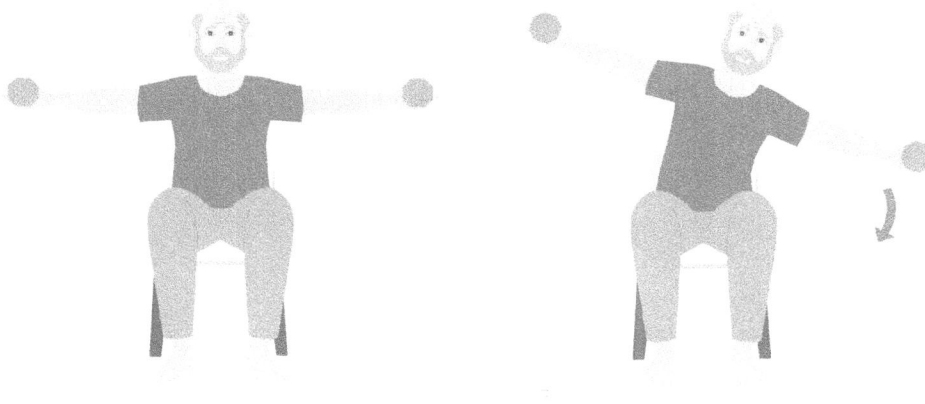

<u>Steps:</u>

1. Position yourself upright in a chair with both feet planted firmly on the ground, creating a stable base. Hold a light weight (a water bottle works great) in each hand to begin. If you have any shoulder or back concerns, consider performing this exercise without weights to ensure safety.

2. Extend your arms to either side, reaching out at shoulder level. This stance not only prepares your muscles for the exercise but also aids in maintaining balance throughout the movement.

3. Gently lean to your left side, guiding the weight towards the floor in a controlled manner. This action targets the obliques, engaging the side core muscles.

4. Smoothly return to your starting position, keeping your movements measured and your core engaged.

5. Repeat the motion on your right side, ensuring an even and balanced workout.

6. Continue to alternate sides, aiming for 10-15 repetitions on each side. This repetition range is designed to effectively work the muscles without overexertion.

Chair Boat Pose

Helps with:	
» **Muscle strengthening** Engages the core muscles, particularly the abdominals and hip flexors, to hold the pose and maintain stability.	» **Improved balance and coordination** Balancing in this pose requires core stabilization and coordination between the upper and lower body.
» **Enhanced joint flexibility** The pose stretches and strengthens the hip flexors and lower back, contributing to better flexibility.	

Safety Precautions:
- Ensure the chair is stable and securely placed on a non-slip surface to prevent any movement. - Keep your spine straight and long throughout the pose to avoid rounding the back, which can put unnecessary pressure on the lower back. - Engage your core muscles actively to support your spine and maintain balance.

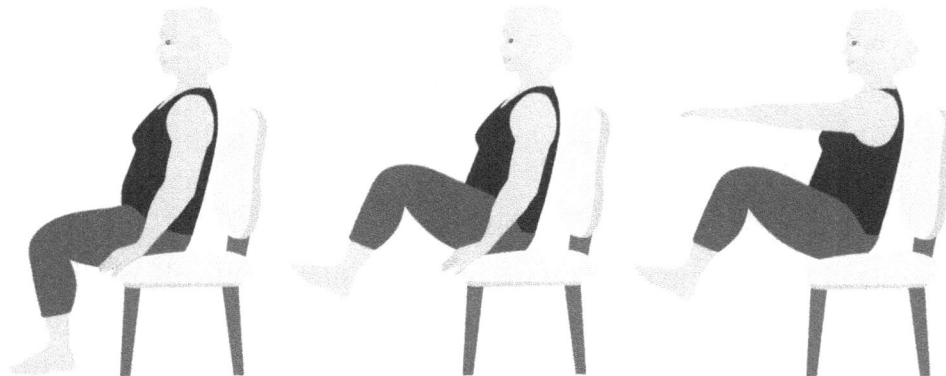

Steps:

1. Start by sitting halfway on a stable chair, feet flat on the floor, and hands resting lightly on the sides of the chair or the seat for support.

2. Engage your core muscles by drawing your navel towards your spine, preparing your body for the lift.

3. Lean slightly back in the chair, keeping your back straight and chest lifted to avoid collapsing the spine.

4. Lift your feet off the floor, bringing your shins parallel to the floor, or as high as comfortable, to initiate the Boat Pose.

5. If possible, release your hands from the chair and extend them forward, parallel to the ground, to increase the engagement of the core muscles. Ensure your shoulders are relaxed and away from your ears.

6. Hold the pose for several breaths, focusing on maintaining balance and stability while keeping the core engaged. The intensity of the pose can be increased by holding it longer or by straightening the legs to form a V shape.

7. To exit the pose, gently lower your feet back to the floor and relax your arms, sitting upright to release the pose.

8. Pause for a moment to observe the effects of the pose before continuing with your practice or moving on with your day.

Chair Supported Warrior II

<table>
<tr><td colspan="2" align="center">Helps with:</td></tr>
<tr>
<td>

» **Muscle strengthening**
This pose strengthens the legs, hips, and core muscles by requiring engagement of the core to maintain stability and support the extended position.

» **Enhanced joint flexibility**
The wide stance stretches the hips and inner thighs, improving flexibility in these areas.

</td>
<td>

» **Improved balance and coordination**
Balancing in this pose with support helps enhance overall stability and coordination.

» **Improved posture**
Engaging the core and aligning the spine in this pose promotes proper posture and spinal alignment.

</td>
</tr>
<tr><td colspan="2" align="center">Safety Precautions:</td></tr>
<tr>
<td colspan="2">

- Ensure proper alignment to avoid strain.
- Avoid if you have hip or knee injuries.

</td>
</tr>
</table>

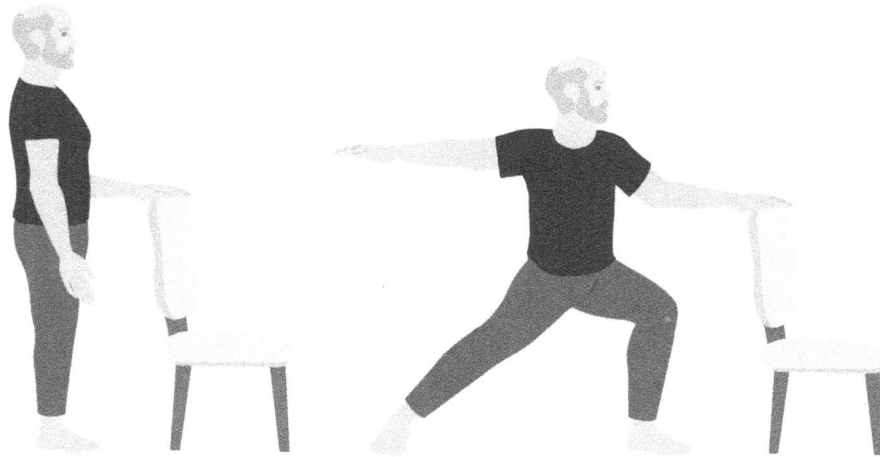

1. Begin by standing behind your chair, using the back for support. This position ensures stability and safety throughout the exercise.

2. Step your feet wide apart, establishing a solid base. Turn your right foot outwards and your left foot to face forward, setting up the foundational stance for Warrior II.

3. Bend your left knee, aiming to align it directly over your ankle. This alignment is crucial for protecting the knee joint and ensuring the exercise's effectiveness.

4. Straighten your right leg, pressing the outer edge of your right foot into the floor for stability. This action engages the leg muscles and helps maintain balance.

5. Extend your right arm back to shoulder height, parallel to the floor, while keeping your left hand on the chair. Turn your head to gaze over your left arm, focusing on a point that helps maintain balance and concentration.

6. Hold this position for several deep breaths, feeling the strength and stretch in your legs and arms. This hold is vital for building stamina and improving concentration.

7. Carefully release the pose and switch sides, repeating the steps with your right leg bent and your left arm extended to ensure a balanced workout.

Chair Plank

Helps with:	
» **Muscle strengthening** This pose engages the core, arms, and shoulders, building overall upper body and core strength.	» **Reduced muscle tension** Engaging and stabilizing the muscles helps release tension in the upper body.

» **Improved balance and coordination**	» **Enhanced joint flexibility**
Holding the plank requires stabilization from multiple muscle groups, enhancing overall balance and coordination.	The pose helps maintain flexibility in the wrists, shoulders, and hips through sustained engagement and support.

Safety Precautions:

- Perform near a wall or stable surface for additional support if needed.
- Avoid if you have shoulder or wrist pain.

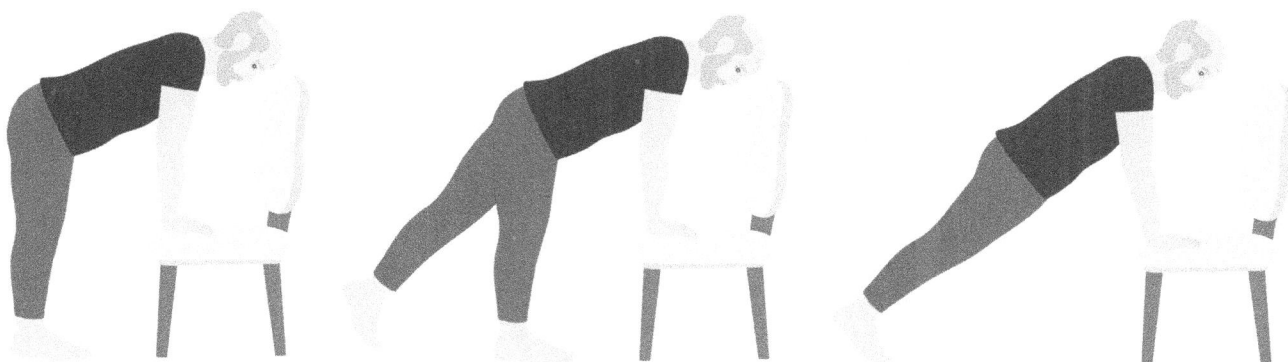

Steps:

1. Start by placing a stable chair against a wall if needed to ensure it won't move during the exercise.

2. Stand facing the chair, keeping your back straight bend forward from the hips, and place both hands on the seat slightly wider than shoulder-width apart. Ensure your wrists are directly under your shoulders.

3. Step back one foot at a time, extending your legs fully behind you, coming onto the balls of your feet. Your body should form a straight line from your head to your heels, similar to the alignment in a traditional plank pose but elevated.

4. Tighten your abdominal muscles and draw your navel towards your spine to keep your core engaged. This supports your lower back and enhances the strength-building aspect of the plank.

5. Hold the plank position, focusing on maintaining a strong, stable posture. Your gaze should be down and slightly forward to keep your neck in a neutral position.

6. Start with holding the pose for 10-30 seconds, gradually increasing the time as your strength improves.

7. Gently step your feet forward towards the chair, and stand up straight to exit the pose.

Enhancing your core strength through chair yoga is a powerful way to improve your overall stability, balance, and functional mobility. By regularly practicing these exercises, you'll find that everyday tasks become easier, your posture improves, and your risk of falls decreases. Remember, the key to success is consistency. Incorporate these poses into your daily routine, listen to your body, and gradually build your strength over time.

A strong core is about creating a solid foundation for all your movements, supporting your spine, and maintaining your independence as you age. Embrace these chair yoga exercises, and you'll be well on your way to a stronger, healthier, and more confident you.

CHAPTER 3
CHAIR YOGA FOR UPPER BODY STRENGTH

As we age, keeping our muscles strong becomes more important than ever. Strong muscles support our joints, keep us mobile, and help prevent falls and injuries. By focusing on exercises that build and maintain muscle strength, we can make daily tasks easier and more enjoyable, from lifting groceries to reaching for items on a high shelf or opening different kinds of medication bottles.

These exercises are designed to be accessible and effective for seniors, promoting gradual progress and lasting strength. By adding these movements to your regular routine, you'll notice increased muscle flexibility and resilience. This chapter emphasizes not only the physical benefits of muscle strengthening but also the boost in confidence and independence that comes with it, helping you lead a more active and fulfilling life.

Upper body strength is essential for maintaining the ability to perform many daily activities independently. The muscles in your arms, shoulders, chest, and upper back are involved in virtually every movement you make, from lifting objects to pushing doors open.

Think about the tasks you perform—changing your bed sheets, reaching for something on a high shelf, or even hugging a loved one. These actions all rely on upper body strength. Here's how your upper body muscles play a role in everyday tasks:

» **Lifting and Carrying**: Whether it's groceries, laundry, or even grandchildren, strong arm and shoulder muscles make lifting and carrying easier and safer.

» **Reaching and Stretching**: Activities like reaching for items on high shelves or stretching to clean windows require strength and flexibility in your upper body.

» **Pushing and Pulling**: From opening heavy doors to pulling a chair closer, these movements engage your chest, back, and arm muscles.

» **Posture and Stability**: A strong upper body supports good posture, reducing the strain on your spine and preventing back and neck pain.

By strengthening your upper body, you enhance your ability to perform these tasks with greater ease and confidence, which improves your overall quality of life.

UPPER BODY STRENGTHENING POSES

Seated Arm Circles

Helps with:	
» **Muscle strengthening** Engages and strengthens the shoulder muscles and upper arms through controlled circular movements.	» **Improved mobility** Enhances flexibility and range of motion in the shoulder joints.
Safety Precautions:	
- Keep your movements slow and controlled to avoid any strain on your shoulders. - If you experience any pain or discomfort, reduce the size of your circles or take a break.	

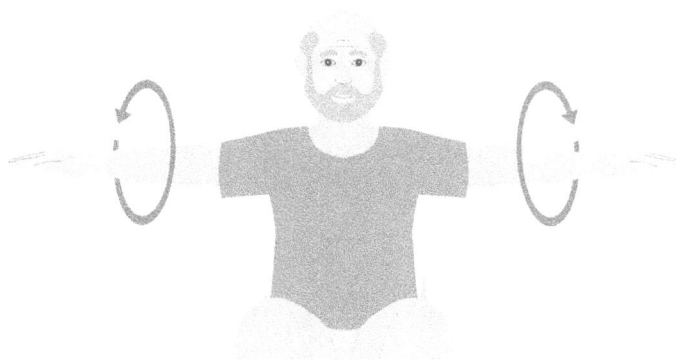

1. Begin by sitting upright in a chair, with your feet flat on the ground.

2. Extend your arms out to the sides at shoulder height, keeping them straight. Ensure your palms are facing down to start, positioning your body in a T-shape.

3. Start making small circles with your arms, moving them in a forward motion. Focus on keeping the circles controlled and your arms level with your shoulders.

4. Gradually increase the size of the circles as you become more comfortable, ensuring you maintain control and do not strain your shoulder muscles.

5. After 15 seconds or when you're ready, reverse the direction of your circles, moving your arms in a backward motion. This change in direction helps to engage different muscles in your shoulders and upper back.

6. Continue performing the arm circles for a total of 30 seconds to 1 minute, alternating between forward and backward motions. You can adjust the duration based on your comfort and fitness level.

7. As you perform the arm circles, remember to breathe deeply and evenly. Proper breathing enhances oxygen flow to your muscles and helps keep you relaxed and focused.

Seated Chest Opener

Helps with:	
» **Muscle strengthening** Stretches and strengthens the chest and shoulder muscles, promoting better upper body strength.	» **Improved posture** Helps counteract the effects of slouching and improves overall posture by opening the chest.
Safety Precautions:	
- Avoid overextending your back. - If you have lower back issues, proceed cautiously.	

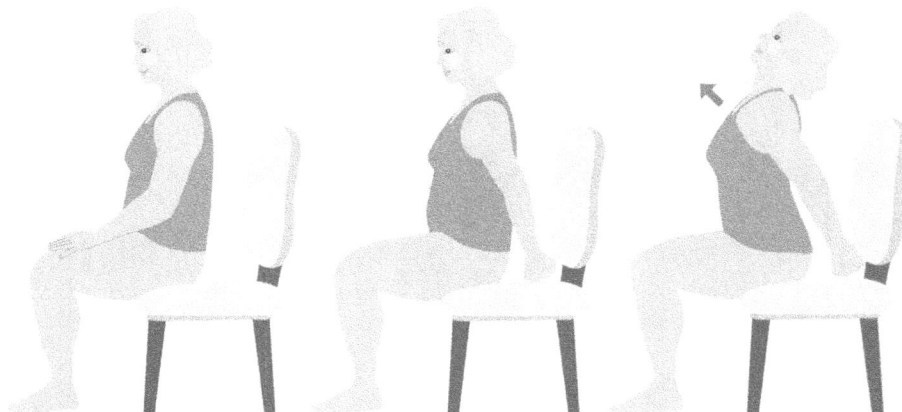

1. Begin by sitting upright in a chair with your feet firmly planted on the floor. This stable position ensures proper alignment and support throughout the exercise.

2. Clasp your hands behind your back. This action prepares your upper body for the stretch and helps in engaging the correct muscles.

3. Inhale deeply, and as you exhale, gently pull your clasped hands downwards. Simultaneously, open your chest and lift your gaze slightly upwards. This movement stretches the chest and shoulders, encouraging a natural opening of the upper body.

4. Hold this position for several breaths, allowing the stretch to deepen with each exhale. The focus should be on maintaining a gentle stretch that opens the chest without straining the back.

5. Carefully release the stretch and relax. The controlled return to a relaxed state helps in maximizing the benefits of the stretch while ensuring safety.

Seated Clapping Hands

Helps with:	
» **Muscle strengthening** Engages the pectoral muscles, shoulders, and upper arms, enhancing upper body strength.	» **Improved coordination** Promotes better hand-eye coordination and arm movement.
Safety Precautions:	
- Clap at a comfortable pace to avoid straining your wrists. - Ideal for those looking for a gentle upper body exercise.	

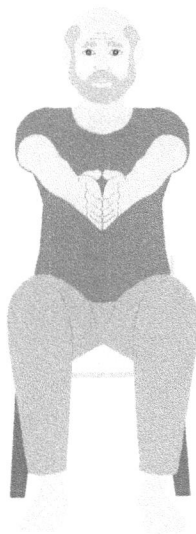

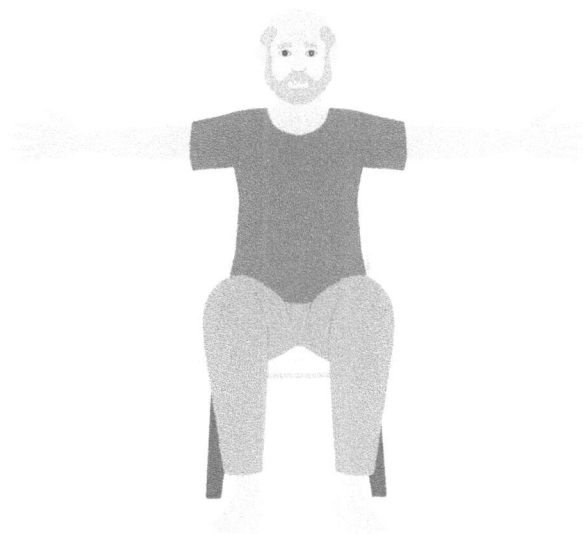

1. Begin by sitting upright in a chair, ensuring your feet are flat on the ground for stability.
2. Extend your arms in front of you at shoulder height, preparing your upper body for the exercise.
3. Bring your hands together in a clap, then open them wide as if embracing the space around you. This motion encourages blood flow and engages the muscles in your arms and shoulders.
4. Continue this clapping motion in a rhythmic manner for 30 seconds to 1 minute, depending on your comfort level. The goal is to maintain a steady pace that feels energizing without causing strain on your wrists or arms.

Chair Upper Body Twists with Arms Extended

Helps with:	
» **Muscle strengthening** Engages the shoulder muscles, upper back, and arms while twisting, promoting strength and flexibility.	» **Core engagement** Strengthens the core muscles, which support upper body movement and stability.
Safety Precautions:	
- Twist gently to avoid straining the spine. - Keep movements controlled and avoid overextending the arms.	

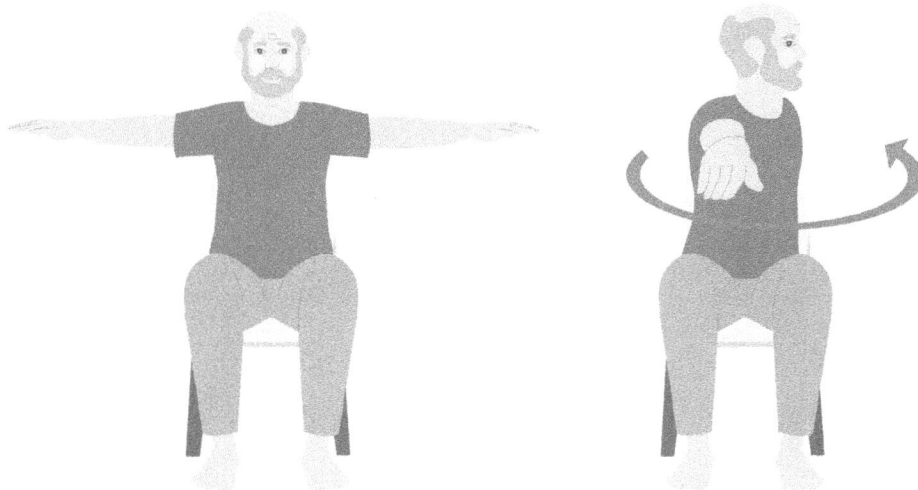

Steps:

1. Begin by sitting upright on a chair with your feet flat on the ground, establishing a stable base.

2. Extend your arms to the sides at shoulder height, creating a T-shape with your body. This position prepares your upper body for the twisting motion.

3. Gently twist your upper body to the left, ensuring your arms remain extended. This movement engages your core and stretches the spine, promoting flexibility.

4. Slowly return to the center before twisting to the right. This alternating pattern ensures an even stretch and strengthening across your body.

5. Continue this sequence for 10-15 repetitions on each side, focusing on controlled movements to maximize benefits and minimize the risk of injury.

Seated Arm Swings

Helps with:	
» **Muscle strengthening** Strengthens the shoulder muscles and upper arms through dynamic swinging movements.	» **Improved circulation** Enhances blood flow to the upper body, promoting muscle health and recovery.
Safety Precautions:	
- Swing your arms gently to avoid shoulder strain. - Ideal for warming up the upper body.	

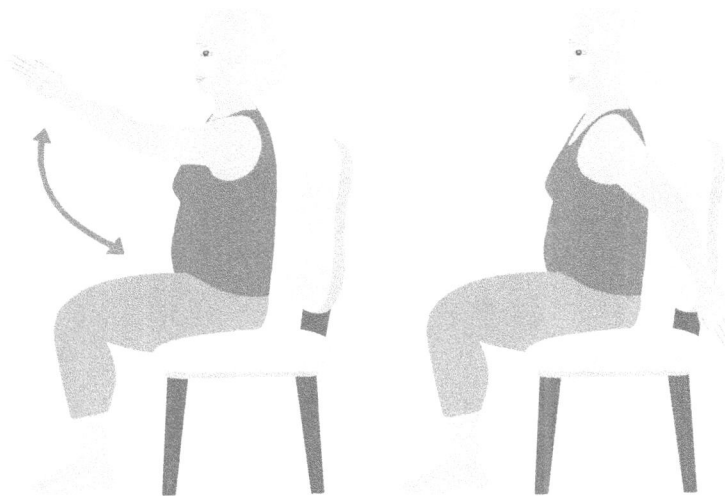

Steps:

1. Sit upright in a chair with your feet flat on the floor, ensuring stability.

2. Allow your arms to hang naturally at your sides. Relax and releasing any tension.

3. Begin by gently swinging your arms forward and upward. As your arms reach shoulder height or slightly higher, keep your movements controlled and fluid.

4. Let your arms swing back and downward, completing the full range of motion.

5. Maintain a natural breathing pattern. Inhale as your arms swing forward and upward, and exhale as they swing back and downward.

6. Continue the arm swings for 30 seconds to 1 minute, depending on your comfort level and fitness. Start with a shorter duration and gradually increase as you build strength and endurance.

Seated Goddess Pose

Helps with:	
» Muscle strengthening Engages and strengthens the shoulder, upper back, and arm muscles by holding the arms in a lifted position.	**» Improved flexibility** Stretches the chest and shoulders, enhancing flexibility and range of motion.
Safety Precautions:	
-Adjust the width of your leg stance to avoid discomfort in the hips or knees. - Keep your spine straight and avoid leaning forward to maintain balance and alignment. - Engage your core throughout the pose for additional support.	

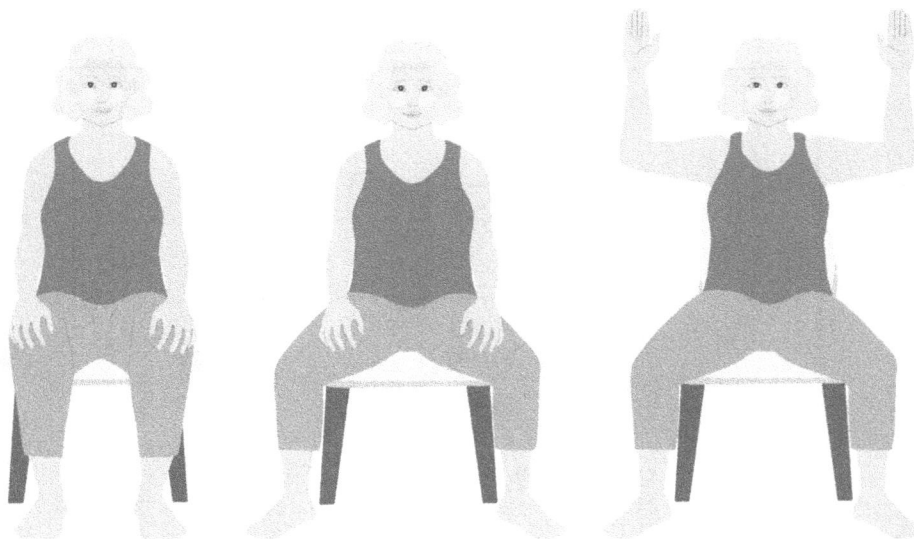

Steps:

1. Sit comfortably towards the front of a stable chair, feet flat on the floor, and spine erect to maintain good posture.

2. Gently open your legs to each side, creating a V-shape with your legs. Adjust the width of your stance to a position that feels comfortable yet provides a gentle stretch in the inner thighs and groin area.

3. Turn your toes slightly outward, in alignment with the direction of your knees, to ensure a natural position that supports hip opening without strain.

4. Activate your abdominal muscles by drawing your navel towards your spine, supporting your upper body and promoting an upright posture.

5. For an added upper body stretch, raise your arms to shoulder height, bending the elbows so your forearms are vertical and palms face forward, resembling the cactus arm position. This can help open the chest and shoulders.

6. Maintain the Goddess Pose, breathing deeply for several breaths. Focus on the sensation of opening in the hips and thighs, and the strength being built in your posture.

7. To release, gently bring your legs back together, returning to the starting position. Lower your arms if they were raised.

8. Take a moment to sit with your feet planted and hands on your lap, breathing deeply to integrate the benefits of the pose.

Chair-Assisted Push-Ups

Helps with:	
» **Muscle strengthening** Targets the chest, shoulders, triceps, and upper back muscles, significantly improving upper body strength.	» **Core engagement** Strengthens the core muscles as they stabilize the body during the push-up movement.
Safety Precautions:	
- Ensure the chair is stable and won't slip. - Keep your core engaged to protect your lower back.	

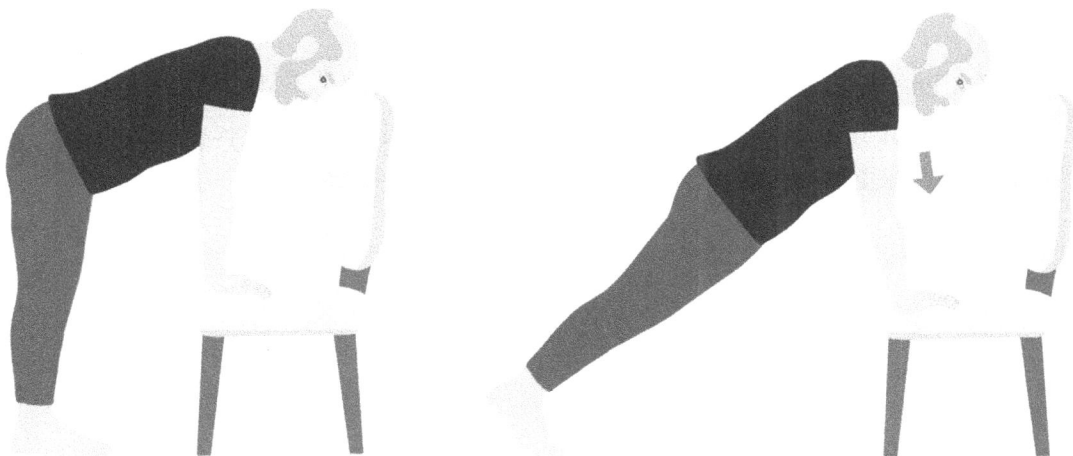

<u>Steps:</u>

1. Begin by standing in front of a stable chair, ensuring it is securely placed against a wall or on a non-slip surface to prevent movement during the exercise.

2. Place your hands on the seat of the chair, positioning them slightly wider than shoulder-width apart. This hand placement allows for a stable base and targets the upper body muscles effectively.

3. Step your feet back until your body is in a plank position, with your weight evenly distributed between your hands and toes. Keep your body in a straight line from head to heels, engaging your core to support your lower back.

4. Bend your elbows to lower your chest towards the seat of the chair, keeping your elbows close to your body. This motion engages the chest, arms, and shoulders.

5. Push through your hands to lift your body back up to the starting plank position, completing one repetition.

6. Aim for 10-15 repetitions, focusing on maintaining proper form and controlled movements throughout the set.

Incorporating these gentle movements into your routine can make a big difference in your upper body strength, muscle flexibility, and joint health. By practicing these exercises regularly, you'll find that your mobility, stability, and resilience improve.

To take your workout to the next level, consider using resistance bands or light weights with these exercises. This added resistance can help build muscle more effectively and make your workout more challenging as you progress.

Imagine the satisfaction of moving with greater ease and confidence, knowing you're taking proactive steps to improve your well-being. Building and maintaining upper body strength isn't just about physical fitness; it's about feeling empowered to live your life to the fullest.

With a stronger upper body, daily tasks become less of a challenge, allowing you to enjoy your activities without fear of strain or injury. Embrace these chair yoga exercises, and take the next step towards a healthier, safer, and more confident lifestyle.

CHAPTER 4
CHAIR YOGA FOR LOWER BODY STRENGTH

Maintaining lower body strength as we age is crucial for overall mobility, stability, and independence. Strong legs and hips provide the foundation for balance, making it easier to perform daily activities such as walking, climbing stairs, and getting out of a chair. Without adequate lower body strength, we become more susceptible to falls and injuries, which can significantly impact our quality of life.

This chapter focuses on chair yoga exercises designed to strengthen the lower body, making these movements accessible and safe for seniors. These exercises target the muscles in the legs, hips, and glutes, promoting gradual progress and sustained strength. By incorporating these movements into your regular routine, you can enhance your lower body strength, improve balance, and increase your overall physical resilience.

Imagine being able to walk with more confidence and stability, or easily stand up from a seated position without assistance. The exercises in this chapter are tailored to help you achieve greater lower body strength, contributing to your independence and overall well-being.

Lower body strength is essential for maintaining your ability to move freely and safely. The muscles in your legs, hips, and glutes are responsible for supporting your body weight, facilitating movement, and ensuring balance.

Think about the tasks you perform each day—walking around your home, climbing stairs, or standing up from a chair. These actions all rely heavily on the strength of your lower body muscles. Here's how these muscles play a role in everyday tasks:

» **Walking and Mobility**: Strong leg muscles help you walk longer distances with ease and stability.

» **Climbing Stairs**: Powerful thighs and glutes make climbing stairs less strenuous and more manageable.

» **Standing Up and Sitting Down**: Robust lower body strength ensures you can stand up from a seated position and sit down smoothly without losing balance.

» **Balance and Stability**: A strong lower body supports your balance, reducing the risk of falls and injuries.

By strengthening your lower body, you enhance your ability to perform these tasks with greater ease and confidence, improving your overall quality of life.

LOWER BODY STRENGTHENING POSES

Seated Leg Swings

Helps with:	
» **Muscle strengthening** This exercise targets the hip flexors and lower abdominal muscles, building strength in the core and legs.	» **Improved balance and coordination** Swinging the knees enhances coordination and stability in the lower body.
» **Improved circulation** The movement promotes blood flow to the lower extremities, improving overall circulation.	
Safety Precautions:	
- Swing your leg gently to avoid strain. - Ensure the chair is stable.	

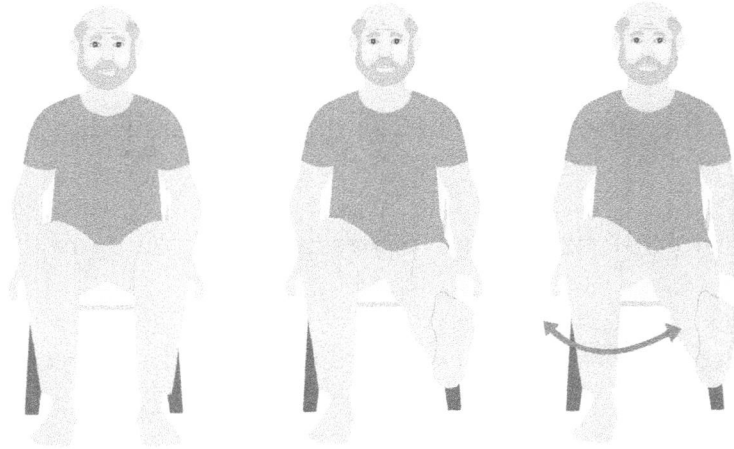

1. Sit at the edge of a stable chair with your feet planted firmly on the floor. This starting position ensures a solid base and prepares your body for movement.

2. Grasp the sides of the chair with both hands for stability. This support is crucial for maintaining balance during the exercise.

3. Extend one leg forward, keeping it as straight as comfortable. This extension prepares your leg for the swinging motion.

4. Gently swing the extended leg from side to side, allowing it to cross in front of your stationary leg. This movement should be controlled and within a comfortable range to avoid strain.

5. Continue the swinging motion for 10-15 repetitions, focusing on smooth, fluid movements to maximize the stretch and mobility benefits.

6. After completing the swings with one leg, pause for a moment to reset, then switch to the other leg, repeating the swinging motion for 10-15 repetitions.

Chair-Assisted Squats

Helps with:	
» **Muscle strengthening** This exercise targets the quadriceps, hamstrings, and glutes, building lower body strength.	» **Improved balance and coordination** Performing squats with chair assistance helps improve balance and stability.

» **Pain reduction**
Strengthening the leg muscles can help alleviate pain in the knees and hips.

Safety Precautions:
- Squat only as low as comfortable.

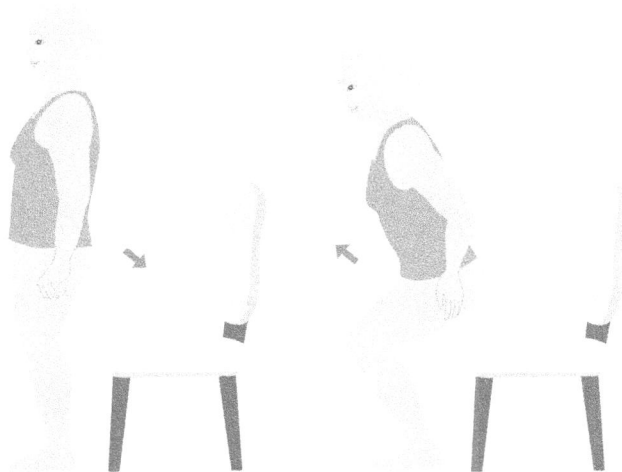

<u>Steps:</u>

1. Begin by standing in front of a stable chair, ensuring it's securely positioned to support you if needed. Your feet should be hip-width apart, aligning your body for optimal movement.
2. Initiate the squat by slowly lowering your body, as if intending to sit down. This movement engages the muscles in your thighs, hips, and buttocks, building strength and flexibility.
3. Bend at the knees and hips, keeping your chest upright and core engaged. This posture ensures a safe, effective squat that targets the right areas without strain.
4. Before making contact with the chair, press through your heels to stand back up. This phase of the exercise challenges your balance and strength, enhancing stability.
5. Aim to complete 10-15 repetitions, maintaining a smooth, controlled motion throughout. Each squat should be performed with care, focusing on form and comfort.

Seated Mountain Climbers

Helps with:	
» **Muscle strengthening**	» **Improved balance and coordination**
Engages and strengthens the quadriceps, hamstrings, and hip flexors through repetitive knee lifts.	The alternating leg movement enhances coordination between the lower body muscles.

» **Enhanced joint flexibility**	» **Improved circulation**
Increases flexibility in the hip and knee joints through dynamic movement.	Promotes blood flow to the lower body, aiding in muscle recovery and overall leg health.

<table>
<tr><td colspan="2" align="center">Safety Precautions:</td></tr>
<tr><td colspan="2">- Move at a pace that is challenging but maintains your balance.
- Ideal for those seeking a cardio workout from a seated position.</td></tr>
</table>

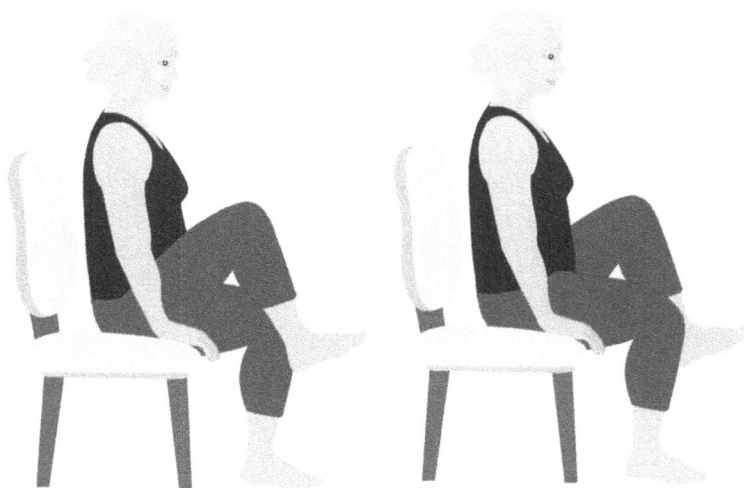

Steps:

1. Begin by sitting at the edge of your chair to allow for greater freedom of movement. Ensure your posture is upright, with your hands resting on the sides of the chair for stability and support.

2. Engage your core muscles as you lift one knee towards your chest, then quickly switch to lift the other knee, creating a motion similar to running. This movement not only strengthens the core but also mobilizes the hip and knee joints.

3. Continue alternating your knees in a brisk but controlled pace. The rapid movement helps to increase your heart rate, providing a cardiovascular workout without the need for standing exercises.

4. Aim to maintain this activity for 30 seconds to 1 minute, depending on your fitness level and comfort. The key is to find a pace that is challenging yet allows you to maintain balance and control throughout the exercise.

Seated Toe Taps

Helps with:	
» **Muscle strengthening** This exercise strengthens the calf muscles, improving lower leg strength. » **Improved balance and coordination** Strengthening the calves enhances stability and coordination in the lower body.	» **Improved circulation** The up-and-down motion promotes blood flow to the lower legs and feet.
Safety Precautions:	
- Tap gently to avoid jarring your legs. - Suitable for those with limited lower body mobility.	

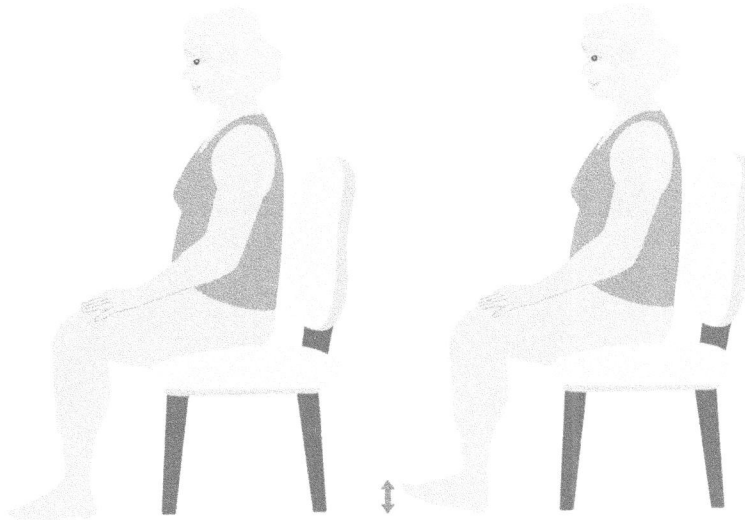

Steps:

1. Position yourself upright in a chair, ensuring your feet are placed flat on the ground. This posture ensures stability and alignment as you perform the toe taps.

Engage your leg muscles to lift your toes while keeping your heels firmly planted on the floor. This action begins the strengthening and circulation enhancement in the lower legs. Gently tap your toes back down to the floor, creating a rhythmic motion. The tapping not only strengthens the muscles but also promotes coordination and agility in the feet and calves. Continue this tapping motion for 20-30 seconds, maintaining a steady pace. Focus on the movement of lifting and lowering the toes, ensuring each tap is controlled and deliberate. Throughout the exercise, keep your posture upright and your movements smooth to maximize the benefits and minimize any risk of strain.

Chair High Lunge

Helps with:	
» **Muscle strengthening** This pose opens up the chest and shoulders, helping to alleviate pain and discomfort in these areas.	» **Improved balance and coordination** Stretching the chest and shoulder muscles helps release tightness and reduce muscle tension.
» **Improved posture** Engaging the core and maintaining proper alignment helps improve overall posture.	

Safety Precautions:
- Ensure the chair is stable. - Avoid this pose if you have severe knee or hip pain.

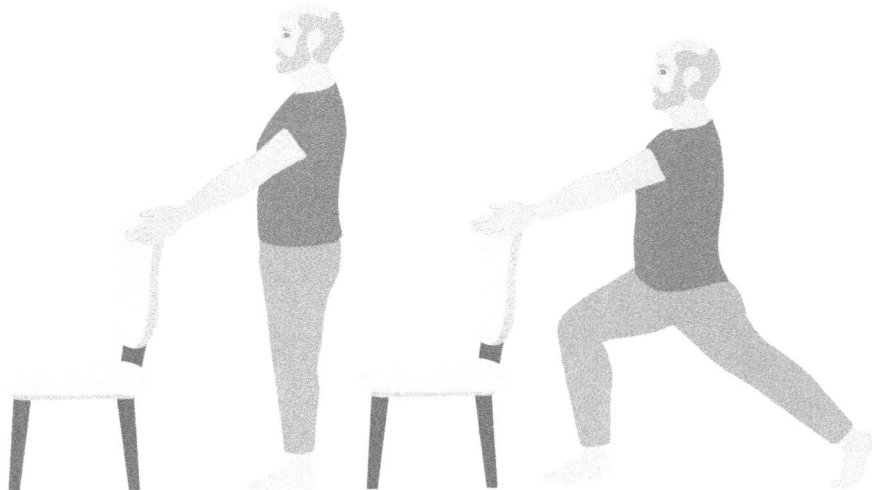

Steps:

1. Position yourself behind the chair, using the backrest as a support to ensure stability throughout the exercise.

2. Take a confident step backward with your left foot, bending your right knee to form a lunge. Your left leg should remain extended behind you, with the heel off the ground, creating a dynamic stretch.

3. Maintain an upright torso and ensure your hips are squared forward, aligning your body for maximum benefit.

4. Stay in this pose for a few deep breaths, feeling the strength in your legs and the stretch in your hips.

5. Gently release and switch legs, repeating the process to ensure balanced strength and flexibility across both sides of your body.

Chair Assisted Leg Lifts

Helps with:	
» **Muscle strengthening** This exercise targets the quadriceps, building strength in the thigh muscles.	» **Improved joint flexibility** Extending and bending the knee enhances flexibility in the knee joint.
» **Pain reduction** Strengthening the muscles around the knee can help reduce pain and improve joint stability.	

Safety Precautions:
- Move slowly and control the movement.   - Do not overextend if you have knee problems.

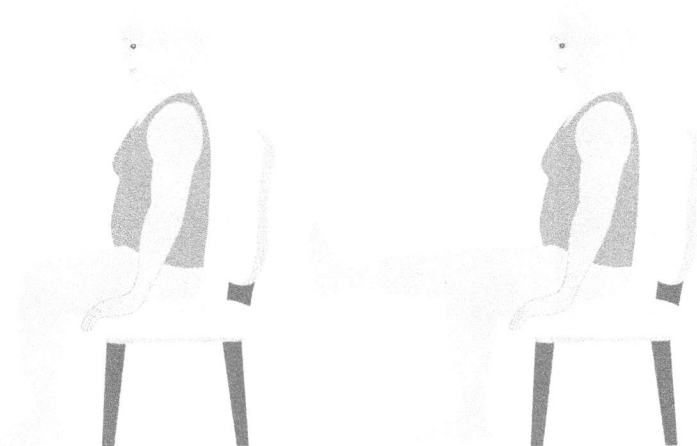

Steps:

1. Begin by sitting upright in a stable chair, ensuring your feet are flat on the ground. This starting position promotes good posture and prepares your body for the exercise.

2. Grasp the sides of the chair lightly for support. This not only aids in maintaining balance during the exercise but also ensures safety and control.

3. Carefully extend one leg out in front of you, striving to keep it parallel to the floor. The goal is to activate the muscles in your thigh and core without straining them.

4. Hold this extended position for a few seconds, focusing on engaging the thigh muscles while keeping the rest of your body stable.

5. Gently lower the leg back to the starting position, controlling the movement to maximize the exercise's benefits.

6. Perform 5-10 repetitions with each leg, alternating to ensure balanced strength and flexibility in both legs.

Seated Bicycle Crunches

<table>
<tr><td colspan="2" align="center"><u>Helps with:</u></td></tr>
<tr>
<td>

» **Muscle strengthening**
This exercise engages the core muscles, including the abdominals and obliques, building overall core strength.

» **Improved posture**
Strengthening the core supports proper spinal alignment, promoting better posture.

</td>
<td>

» **Improved balance and coordination**
Coordinating the leg and core movements enhances stability and coordination.

</td>
</tr>
<tr><td colspan="2" align="center"><u>Safety Precautions:</u></td></tr>
<tr><td colspan="2">

- Move in a controlled manner to avoid strain on the lower back.
- Not recommended for those with acute lower back pain.

</td></tr>
</table>

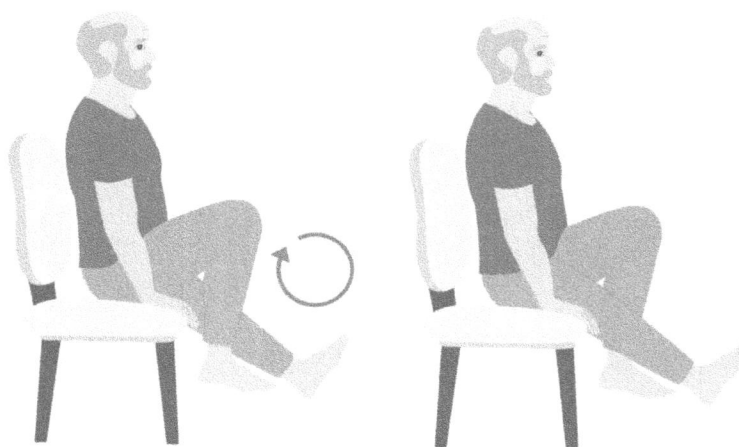

<u>Steps:</u>

1. Sit at the edge of a stable chair, leaning back slightly with hands gripping the sides for support. This starting position helps maintain balance and ensures safety throughout the exercise.

2. Gently lift your feet off the ground, engaging your core to stabilize your body.

3. Simulate a cycling motion by alternately bringing one knee towards your chest and extending the other leg forward. This movement should be performed smoothly and at a comfortable pace to avoid any strain.

4. Continue this pedaling action for 30 seconds to 1 minute. Focus on maintaining a steady rhythm, which helps with coordination and keeps the core engaged without overexertion.

By regularly practicing these chair yoga exercises, you can build and maintain lower body strength, which is crucial for everyday activities and overall mobility. These movements will help you enhance your balance, reduce the risk of falls, and support joint health. With increased lower body strength, you'll find it easier to move confidently and independently, contributing to a more active and fulfilling lifestyle.

Imagine the satisfaction of being able to walk longer distances, stand up with ease, and move about your day without worrying about losing your balance. By dedicating time to these exercises, you are investing in your strength and independence, empowering yourself to enjoy life to the fullest.

With these chair yoga exercises, you are taking a proactive step towards a stronger, healthier, and more independent you. Embrace these movements, and let them guide you to a more confident and active lifestyle. You've got this!

CHAPTER 5
CHAIR YOGA FOR BALANCE AND COORDINATION

As we age, maintaining stability and balance becomes crucial for preventing falls and ensuring overall mobility. Falls can lead to serious injuries that significantly impact a senior's quality of life and independence. That's why this chapter is dedicated to exercises designed to improve your stability, balance, and strength. These chair yoga exercises are tailored to help you develop better coordination and muscle strength, giving you the confidence to move through your daily activities safely and with ease.

Improving your balance and stability is directly connected to building your overall strength. When you work on your balance, you engage your core, leg, and upper body muscles, which in turn enhances your strength. Strong muscles support your joints, maintain proper alignment, and provide the foundation needed for stable movements.

Imagine being able to carry a basket of laundry up the stairs, bend down to tie your shoes, or step out of the shower without the fear of slipping. Envision yourself confidently stepping onto a bus or into a car, navigating uneven sidewalks, or lifting your grandchild with ease. Improved balance and stability can make all these tasks feel much safer and more manageable.

Balance and coordination are essential for maintaining mobility and preventing falls. Think about the daily activities that require balance and coordination—walking, standing up, reaching for objects, or even navigating around furniture. These actions all rely on your ability to balance and coordinate your movements effectively. Here's how balance and coordination play a role in everyday tasks:

» **Walking**: Strong balance helps you walk steadily, preventing trips and falls.

» **Standing Up**: Good coordination allows you to transition smoothly from sitting to standing without losing balance.

» **Reaching and Bending**: Whether you're reaching for something on a high shelf or bending down to pick something up, balance and coordination keep you steady and safe.

» **Navigating Spaces**: Moving around your home or in public spaces with confidence requires solid balance and coordination.

By improving your balance and coordination, you enhance your ability to perform these tasks with greater ease and confidence, which significantly boosts your quality of life.

BALANCE AND COORDINATION POSES

Seated Dancer Pose

Helps with:	
» **Improves balance and coordination** It strengthens the legs and core muscles, improving overall lower body strength.	» **Strengthens the legs and core** Engaging the core and maintaining alignment of the spine helps our posture.
Safety Precautions:	
- Be cautious to maintain balance. - Avoid if you have knee or shoulder injuries.	

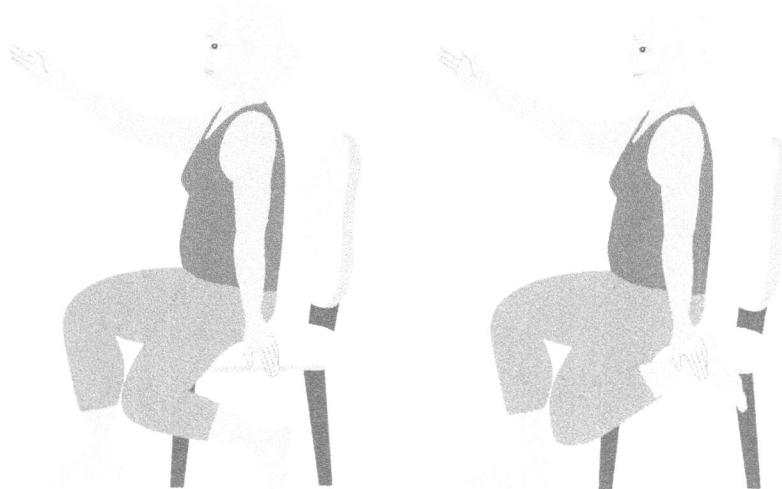

Steps:

1. Start by sitting upright on the side of your chair, ensuring your feet are flat on the floor for a stable base.

2. Bend your left knee and grasp the outside of your left foot or ankle with your left hand. This action initiates the stretch and prepares your body for the pose.

3. Apply a gentle press with your foot against your hand while extending the leg slightly behind you. This extension opens up the thigh and shoulder, deepening the stretch.

4. For additional balance, extend your right arm forward or use the chair for stability. This helps maintain your balance and enhances the overall effectiveness of the pose.

5. Hold this position for several breaths, focusing on a steady, even breathing pattern to maximize the pose's benefits.

6. After holding, gently release and switch sides to ensure a balanced stretch across both sides of the body.

Chair Supported Warrior Flow

Helps with:	
» **Improved balance and coordination** The flowing sequence of movements between different warrior poses challenges stability and enhances coordination, requiring continuous engagement of core and leg muscles.	» **Muscle strengthening** Transitioning through warrior poses strengthens the legs, hips, and core, providing better support and stability for the body.
» **Enhanced joint flexibility** The movements stretch and mobilize the hips, knees, and ankles, improving joint flexibility and range of motion.	» **Improved posture** Engaging the core and maintaining proper alignment during the flow promotes better posture and spinal alignment.
Safety Precautions:	
- Move smoothly between poses to avoid strain. - Use the chair for support throughout the flow.	

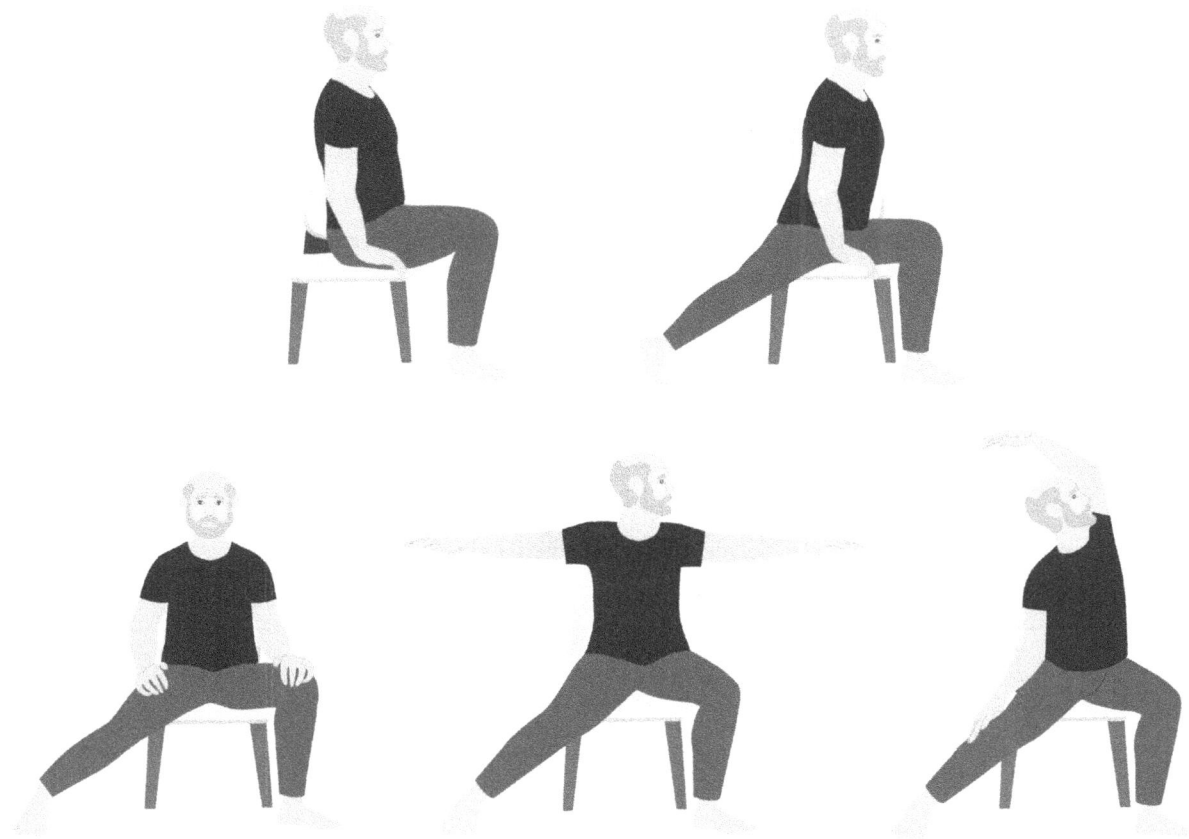

Steps:

1. Begin by sitting at the edge of your chair, turning your legs and body to the left side, ensuring it's stable.

2. Inhale deeply and step your right foot back into a high lunge, positioning the back straight up to the sky and bending the front knee to align over the front ankle. This posture starts the engagement and strengthening of your legs.

3. Smoothly transition into Warrior II by rotating your back foot flat and opening your hips and chest sideways. Extend your arms parallel to the floor, shoulder height, gazing over your front hand. This pose enhances leg strength and opens the hips and chest.

4. For the Reverse Warrior, keep the front knee bent, lift your front arm towards the ceiling, and let your back hand gently rest on the back leg. This action stretches the side of the body, improving flexibility in the spine and sides.

5. After holding the pose for a few breaths, smoothly transition to the other side, repeating the sequence. This balance ensures even strength and flexibility development on both sides of the body.

6. Continue alternating sides for several cycles, moving with your breath. This repetition helps to deepen the poses with each cycle, promoting flexibility and strength.

Chair Supported Chair Tree

Helps with:	
» **Improved balance and coordination** This pose helps enhance stability and coordination by challenging your balance while using a chair for support.	» **Muscle strengthening** It strengthens the legs and core muscles, improving overall lower body strength.
» **Improved posture** Engaging the core and maintaining proper alignment of the spine helps improve overall posture.	

Safety Precautions:
- Keep your foot away from the knee joint to avoid pressure.   - Maintain a straight spine to prevent strain.

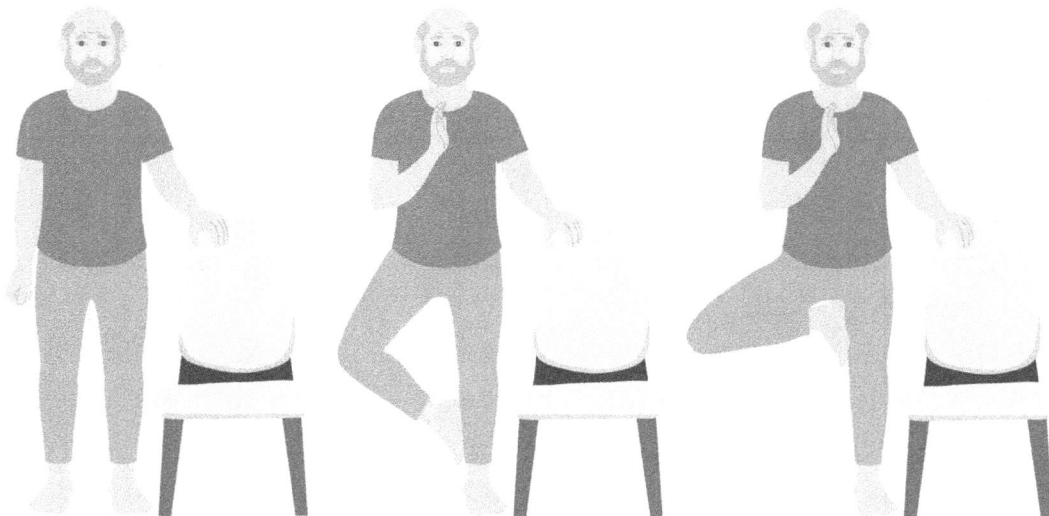

Steps:

1. Begin by standing beside your chair, using one hand to lightly hold onto the backrest for support. This touchpoint is your grounding, ensuring stability as you find your balance.

2. Carefully place your right foot against your inner left thigh or calf, making sure to avoid placing any pressure on your knee. This mindful placement is key to protecting your joints while engaging the muscles in your leg and core.

3. Elevate your right hand to a prayer position at your chest or reach it skyward, creating a line of energy that extends through your entire body. This gesture is not just about balance; it's a symbol of unity and focus.

4. Hold this position for several deep, calming breaths, allowing yourself to fully immerse in the moment. Feel the strength in your standing leg and the steadiness of your breath.

5. Gently release and switch sides, offering your body the same attention and care.

Chair Assisted Standing Back Arch

Helps with:	
» **Improves balance and coordination** Balancing while arching the back with chair support enhances stability.	» **Strengthens the core and back muscles** Engages the lower back and abdominal muscles, improving overall balance.
Safety Precautions:	
- Use the chair for support and avoid over-arching your back. - Not recommended for those with severe back pain.	

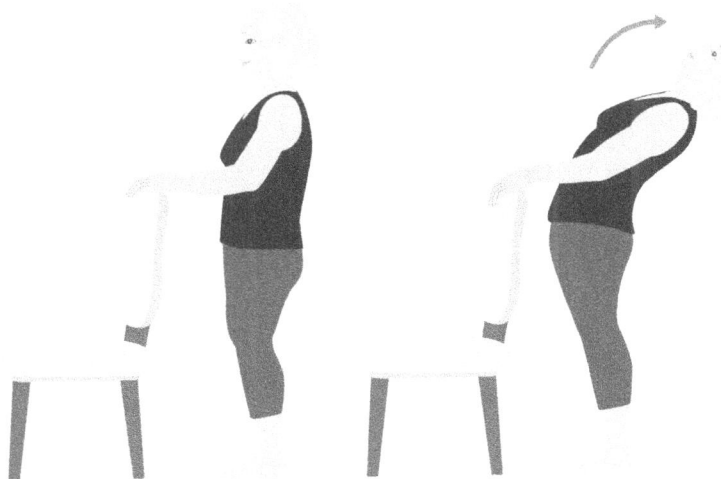

Steps:

1. Begin by positioning yourself behind the chair, ensuring it is stable. Grasp the backrest with both hands for support.

2. Inhale deeply, and as you exhale, gently arch your back. Engage in pushing your hips slightly forward while simultaneously lifting your chest towards the ceiling. This movement encourages a graceful extension of the spine and opens the front of the body.

3. Maintain this arched position for a few deep breaths. Focus on the sensation of expansion across your chest and the gentle strengthening of your back muscles. Ensure to keep the movement within a comfortable range to avoid any strain.

4. To conclude, inhale and gently return to a neutral standing position. Take a moment to observe any shifts in your body, perhaps noticing a newfound sense of openness across the chest and back.

Chair Half Moon Balance

Helps with:	
» **Improves balance and coordination** Balancing while extending one leg and arm challenges stability and coordination.	» **Strengthens the core and legs** Engages the core and leg muscles, promoting better balance.

Safety Precautions:
- Use the chair for support to maintain balance. - Avoid if you have balance or lower body mobility issues.

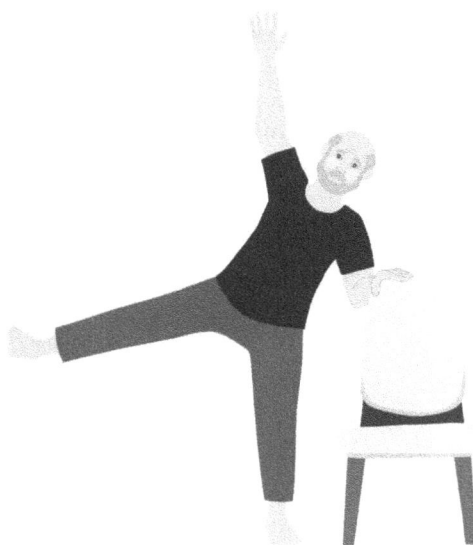

Steps:

1. Begin by standing with your left side next to the chair, placing your left hand on the backrest for support. This ensures stability as you enter the pose.

2. Carefully shift your weight onto your left leg, grounding through the foot for balance. This activates the muscles in the standing leg, preparing them for the pose.

3. Gradually lift your right leg to the side, keeping it straight, while simultaneously tilting your torso to the left. Aim to create a straight line from your left foot through your torso and out through your right fingertips, which are reaching towards the sky.

4. As you balance, extend your right arm upward, directly in line with your left leg. This action not only enhances the stretch along the right side of your body but also encourages a strong sense of balance and alignment.

5. Maintain this position for a few deep, steady breaths, focusing on the stretch and strength being cultivated in the pose.

6. To exit, gently lower your right leg back to the ground and return to a standing position before switching sides to ensure a balanced practice.

Chair Squat Jumps

Helps with:	
» **Muscle strengthening** This dynamic exercise targets the quadriceps, hamstrings, glutes, and calves, significantly enhancing lower body strength.	» **Improved balance and coordination** The explosive movement from the squat to the jump improves overall stability and coordination.
Safety Precautions:	
- Move softly to protect your knees and ankles. - Not recommended for those with severe knee or hip issues.	

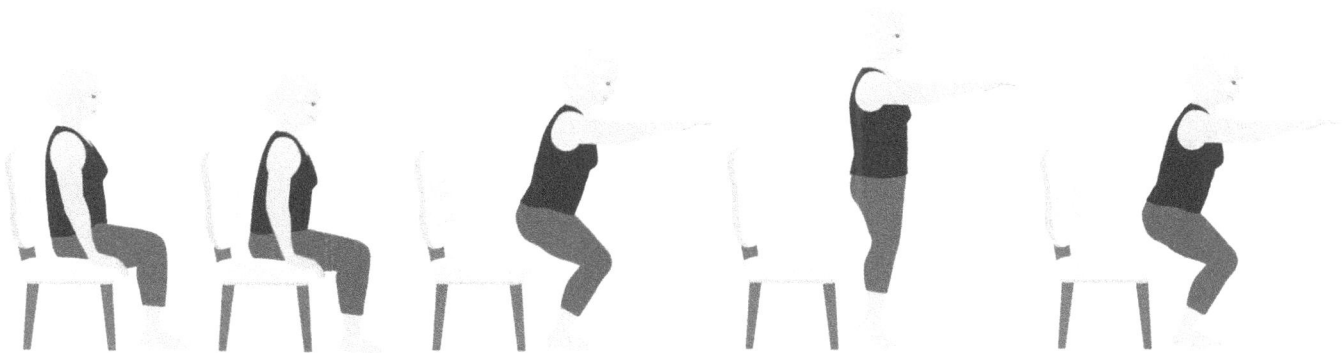

Steps:

1. Begin by sitting halfway on a stable chair with your feet hip-width apart and flat on the floor. Ensure the chair is securely positioned to prevent any movement during the exercise.

2. Lean slightly forward, engaging your core, and press through your heels to stand up from the chair. As you reach a standing position, extend your arms in front of you for balance.

3. Instead of performing an explosive jump, raise onto the balls of your feet, lifting your heels off the ground. This motion mimics the jump's upward phase, activating the calf muscles and glutes with minimal impact on the joints.

4. Reverse the motion by lowering your heels back to the floor and then slowly bending your knees to return to a seated position on the chair. This controlled descent is crucial for building strength in the thighs and glutes.

5. To add a slight cardiovascular challenge without the impact of a traditional jump, quickly stand again and repeat the heel raise. This rapid succession of movements will help increase your heart rate.

6. Perform 10-15 repetitions of this modified squat to heel raise, focusing on smooth transitions between sitting and standing to maintain balance and engage the targeted muscle groups effectively.

Chair Supported Sun Salutation

Helps with:	
» **Improves balance and coordination** The sequence of movements enhances coordination and stability.	» **Strengthens the core and legs** Engages multiple muscle groups, promoting better balance and strength.
Safety Precautions:	

- Keep your movements smooth and controlled to avoid any strain, particularly when transitioning.
- Adjust the depth of the poses to your comfort level, especially in forward folds and lunges, to prevent overstretching.

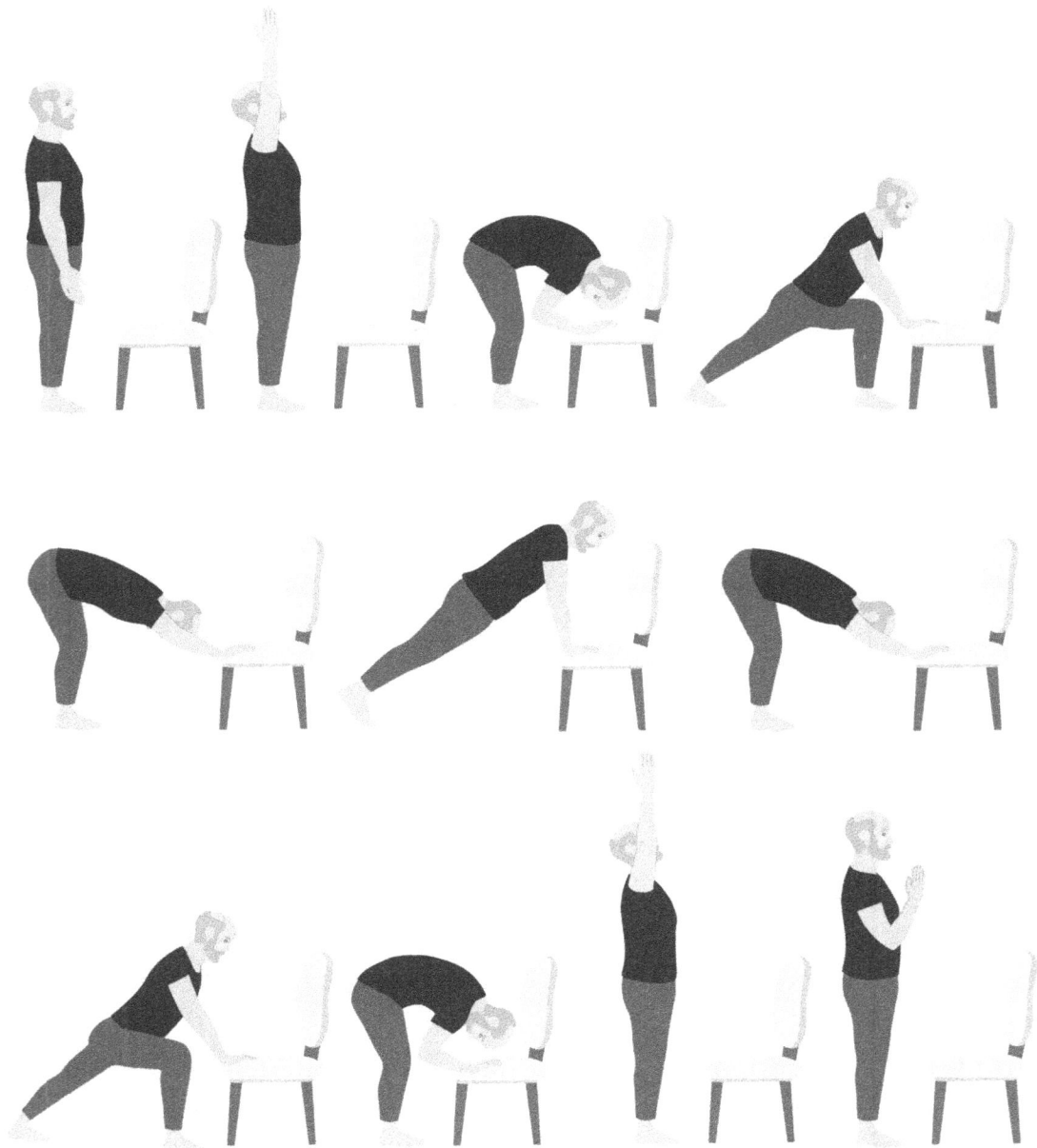

Steps:

1. Stand in front of your chair, facing the seat, with arms by your side and feet hip-distance apart. This is your starting position.

2. Inhale and reach your arms up towards the sky, elongating your spine and stretching your entire body.

3. As you exhale, fold forward, bending your knees slightly. Place your hands on the chair seat, letting your head drop to relax your neck and shoulders.

4. Inhale and step your right foot back into a modified Warrior I pose. Keep your left knee bent directly above your left ankle, hips facing forward. Place your hands on the chair for support, lengthening through the spine.

5. Exhale and step your left foot back to join your right, coming into a Downward Dog position with your hands still on the chair. Allow your head to drop between your arms, pulling your hips back.

6. Engage your core and shift your upper body forward into a Plank position, shoulders stacked over your wrists, keeping your body in a straight line supported by the chair.

7. Inhale, and as you exhale, return to your Downward Dog position, extending your arms and pulling your hips back.

8. Step your right foot forward under your chair, returning to a modified Warrior I pose on the opposite side. Take a few breaths in this position.

9. As you exhale, step your left foot forward to meet your right, returning to a forward fold with your hands on the chair, head dropped, and knees bent.

10. Inhale, bend your knees slightly, and with a strong push through your legs, bring yourself back up, sweeping your arms up towards the sky.

11. Exhale and bring your hands to your heart, taking a moment to breathe and prepare to repeat the sequence, this time stepping your left foot back first.

By regularly practicing these chair yoga exercises, you can significantly improve your coordination, strength, and confidence. These movements will help you enhance your balance and stability, reducing the risk of falls and ensuring safer daily activities. As you build your strength and balance, you will find it easier to perform everyday tasks, such as walking, standing, and reaching, with greater ease and assurance.

Imagine the peace of mind that comes with knowing you can move confidently and securely throughout your day. Improved balance and coordination are essential for maintaining your independence and enjoying a more active, fulfilling lifestyle. By dedicating time to these exercises, you are investing in your strength and stability, empowering yourself to enjoy life to the fullest. Embrace these chair yoga exercises and take a proactive step towards a safer, more confident, and more independent you. You've got this!

CHAPTER 6
CHAIR YOGA FOR FLEXIBILITY AND MOBILITY

Improving flexibility and mobility is essential as we age to maintain overall physical health and enhance our quality of life. Stiffness in joints and muscles can make everyday activities, such as bending, reaching, and walking, more difficult and uncomfortable. This chapter focuses on chair yoga exercises designed to increase flexibility and mobility, making daily movements easier and more fluid.

By emphasizing the importance of flexibility and mobility, this chapter provides a variety of chair yoga poses that target different muscle groups and joints. These exercises are designed to be gentle yet effective, allowing seniors to gradually improve their range of motion in a safe and controlled manner. Enhanced flexibility and mobility not only make daily tasks more manageable but also contribute to overall well-being and independence.

Imagine being able to reach for something on a high shelf, bend down to tie your shoes, or simply walk with a greater sense of ease. The exercises in this chapter are tailored to help you achieve greater flexibility and mobility, supporting your ability to perform everyday activities with confidence.

Seated Leg Stretches

Helps with:	
» **Enhanced joint flexibility** This pose stretches the hamstrings, calves, and lower back, improving overall flexibility.	» **Pain reduction** It helps to alleviate lower back and leg pain by stretching tight muscles.
» **Improved circulation** Stretching the legs promotes blood flow to the lower extremities.	» **Better muscle elasticity** Regular practice improves the elasticity of the muscles and connective tissues.

Safety Precautions:

- Do not overstretch; go only as far as comfortable.
- Avoid if you have severe sciatica.

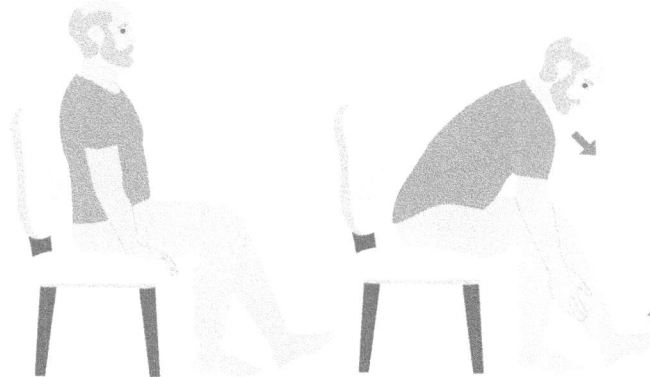

Steps:

1. Start by sitting on the edge of a stable chair, ensuring your posture is upright. This initial position helps maintain balance and alignment for an effective stretch.

2. Fully extend one leg forward, resting the heel on the ground and toes pointing upwards. If you find it challenging, it's perfectly fine to keep a slight bend in the knee. This position targets the hamstring and calf of the extended leg.

3. Keep the other foot flat on the floor to support balance and stability.

4. Inhale deeply to prepare. As you exhale, gently lean forward from your hips towards the extended leg. This forward motion enhances the stretch in the hamstring and lower back. Move into the stretch only as far as comfortable, avoiding any strain.

5. Hold the position for a few breaths, allowing the stretch to deepen gently with each exhale. This not only aids in flexibility but also promotes relaxation.

6. After holding, gently return to the starting position and switch legs, repeating the stretch to ensure balanced flexibility on both sides.

Chair Butterfly Pose

Helps with:	
» **Enhanced joint flexibility** Stretches the hips and inner thighs, enhancing range of motion and increasing flexibility. » **Pain reduction** Relieves tightness and discomfort in the hips and lower back.	» **Improved circulation** Promotes blood flow to the lower body and improves hip mobility.
Safety Precautions:	
- Enter and exit the pose gently to avoid strain on the knees and hips. - Adjust the height of the blocks according to your comfort level, choosing a height that allows you to maintain the pose without discomfort.	

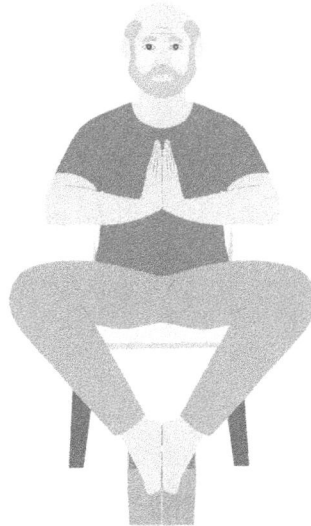

Steps:

1. Prepare Your Space: Sit on a stable chair. If you don't have yoga blocks, consider alternatives like stacked books for firm support, firm pillows or cushions for softer support, sturdy boxes, folded blankets or towels for adjustable firmness, or robust shoe boxes. Place your chosen support on the floor in front of the chair, adjusting to a height that suits your flexibility—typically, the lowest or medium setting for most.

2. Sit towards the chair's front and bring the soles of your feet together, knees falling to the sides into the butterfly position. Place each foot on your chosen support, ensuring stability.

3. Sit tall to lengthen your spine, bring your hands to your heart in a prayer pose or hold your knees for support and to avoid any strain.

4. Focus on relaxing into the stretch and stay in the position for several deep breaths, aiming for up to a minute or as comfortable. Use each exhale to potentially deepen the relaxation and stretch.

5. To release, carefully lift your knees, remove your feet from the supports, and bring legs together. Set aside the supports.

6. With feet flat on the floor, take a few deep breaths to absorb the pose's benefits.

Seated Jumping Jacks

Helps with:	
» **Muscle strengthening** This exercise engages the core, arms, and legs, building overall body strength.	» **Improved balance and coordination** The dynamic movement improves coordination and stability.
» **Improved circulation** The cardiovascular nature of the exercise promotes blood flow throughout the body.	
Safety Precautions:	
- Move in a controlled manner. - If you have joint issues, be cautious with the movements.	

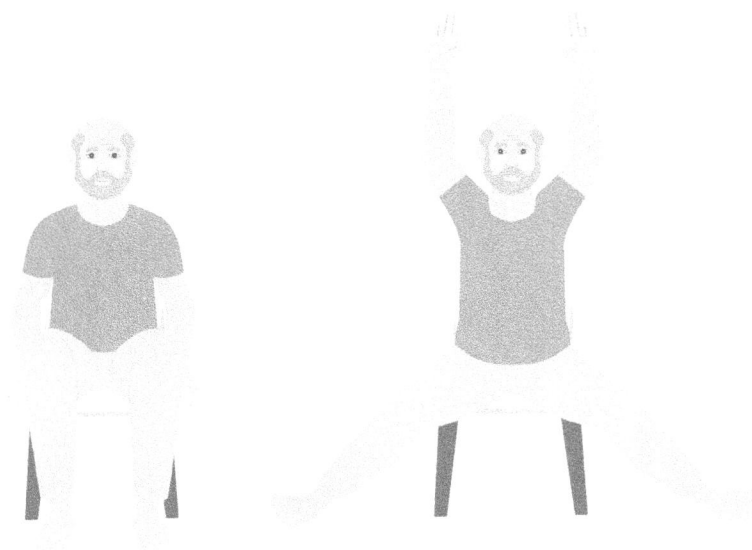

Steps:

1. Begin by sitting upright in a chair, legs together, and arms resting at your sides. Activate your lower abdominal muscles to reduce strain on your back.

2. This starting position ensures stability and readiness for the movement.

3. With a smooth, coordinated motion, extend your legs simultaneously raising your arms above your head. This action mimics the dynamic motion of standing jumping jacks, engaging multiple muscle groups.

4. Carefully return to the starting position, maintaining control and balance throughout the movement. This return phase is crucial for coordinating the exercise and ensuring safety.

5. Aim for 10-20 repetitions, adjusting the number based on your comfort and fitness level. Each repetition should be performed with intention, focusing on controlled movements to maximize benefits while minimizing the risk of strain.

Seated Sphinx Pose

Helps with:	
» **Pain reduction** This pose gently arches the lower back, providing relief from lower back pain by reducing pressure on the spine. » **Improved posture** By encouraging proper spinal alignment, this pose helps improve overall posture.	» **Reduced muscle tension** The gentle extension helps release tightness in the lower back and abdominal muscles.
Safety Precautions:	
- Keep your movements gentle and avoid straining your lower back. - If you have severe back issues, consult a healthcare professional first.	

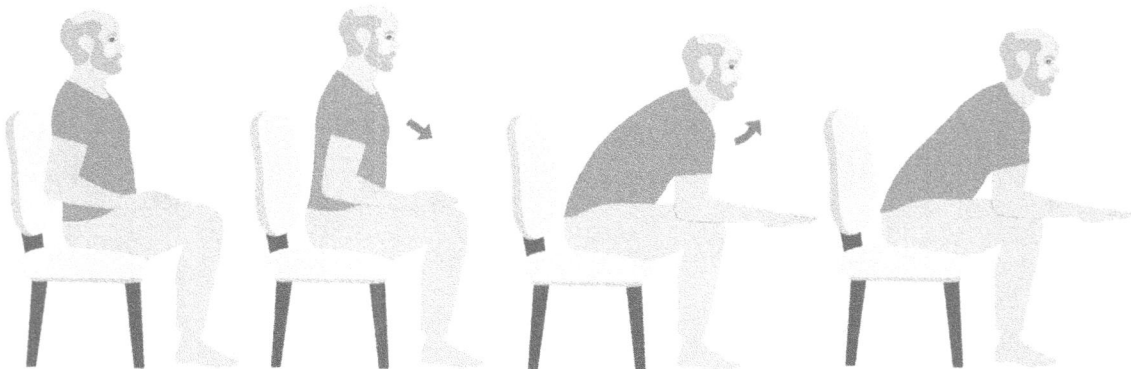

Steps:

1. Position yourself at the front edge of a chair, ensuring your feet are planted firmly on the ground, shoulder-width apart.

2. Initiate the movement by bending forward from your hips, keeping your spine straight to maintain its natural curvature.

3. Slide your hands down your thighs while gently lowering your elbows to rest them on your thighs, transitioning smoothly into the pose.

4. Adjust your position so your elbows are directly beneath your shoulders, forming a 90-degree angle with your arms. This alignment replicates the traditional Sphinx Pose while seated, focusing on spinal integrity and shoulder openness.

5. Slightly lift your chest, creating a gentle arch in your back. This movement emphasizes spinal extension and chest opening, enhancing the stretch.

6. Extend your neck forward, keeping it in line with your spine, to ensure a comprehensive stretch without straining.

7. Hold this position for 5 breaths, focusing on deep, steady inhalations and exhalations to support relaxation and effectiveness of the pose.

8. To conclude, gently raise your torso back to the starting position. Aim for up to 3 repetitions, each time focusing on maintaining smooth movements and proper alignment.

Chair Flutter Kicks

Helps with:	
» **Muscle strengthening** Strengthens the core, hip flexors, and lower abdominal muscles.	» **Improved balance and coordination** Improves overall balance and coordination by engaging the core muscles to maintain stability while performing the kicks.
» **Enhanced joint flexibility** Increases flexibility in the hips and lower body, promoting a greater range of motion.	» **Improved circulation** Promotes blood flow to the lower body, aiding in muscle recovery and overall leg health.
Safety Precautions:	
- Move in a controlled manner to prevent lower back strain. - Suitable for those with a moderate level of abdominal strength.	

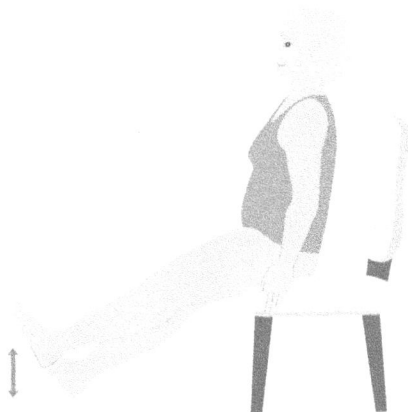

1. Begin by sitting on the edge of a chair. This position allows you to maintain balance and ensures the effectiveness of the exercise. Lean slightly back, but ensure your spine remains aligned to avoid any strain on your back.

2. Hold onto the sides of the chair for support. This grip will help you maintain your balance and position as you perform the flutter kicks.

3. Extend your legs in front of you, raising them slightly off the floor. Keep your legs straight, engaging your core muscles to support the movement.

4. Start to alternately lift each leg in a small, fluttering motion. This action should be controlled and steady, focusing on engaging the lower abdominals and hip flexors with each flutter.

5. Continue the flutter kicks for 30 seconds to 1 minute, depending on your comfort and ability. The goal is to maintain a steady pace and controlled movement throughout the exercise to maximize the benefits while minimizing the risk of strain.

Seated Upward Dog Pose

Helps with:	
» **Enhanced joint flexibility** Stretches the chest, shoulders, and spine, enhancing flexibility in the upper body.	» **Improved spinal mobility** Increases the range of motion in the spine and shoulders, improving overall upper body mobility.
» **Pain reduction** Alleviates tension in the upper back and shoulders, reducing discomfort and promoting relaxation.	
Safety Precautions:	
- Avoid straining your lower back. - If you have severe back issues, consult a healthcare professional first.	

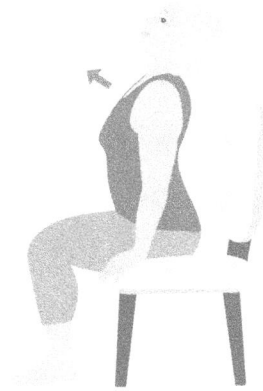

<u>Steps:</u>

1. Position yourself at the edge of your chair, ensuring your feet are solidly grounded.

2. Place your hands on either side of the chair, right beside your hips, ready to lift and support your body.

3. Press down into your hands, engage your core, and lift your chest toward the ceiling, allowing your back to gently arch as you direct your gaze upwards.

4. As you lift, draw your shoulders down and back, away from your ears, to open up the chest fully.

5. Maintain this uplifted posture for a few calming breaths, feeling the stretch across your chest and the strength in your spine.

6. Gently ease back into a neutral sitting position, carrying with you the openness and strength you've cultivated.

Chair Spinal Twist

<u>Helps with:</u>	
» **Enhanced joint flexibility** The Chair Spinal Twist gently stretches the muscles and ligaments along the spine, improving flexibility in the vertebrae and surrounding joints.	» **Improved spinal mobility** By rotating the torso, this pose increases the range of motion in the spine, making it easier to perform daily activities that involve twisting and turning.
» **Pain reduction** The twisting motion helps to alleviate tension in the lower back and can relieve discomfort caused by prolonged sitting or poor posture.	» **Improved posture** Engaging the core and maintaining an upright position during the twist strengthens the muscles that support good posture, helping to prevent back pain and improve overall posture.

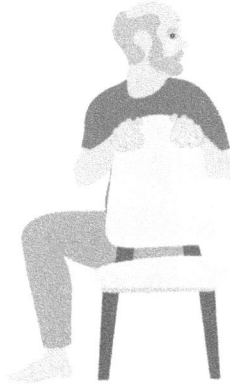

Steps:

1. Begin by sitting sideways on the chair, positioning yourself to face the left. This orientation prepares your body for the twist and ensures a full range of motion.

2. Grasp the back of the chair with both hands, establishing a firm grip that will aid in deepening the twist.

3. Take a deep inhalation to prepare your body. As you exhale, engage your core and twist your torso to the left, using your hands for gentle leverage. Look over your left shoulder to complete the twist, ensuring the movement extends throughout the spine.

4. Hold this position for a few breaths, allowing each exhalation to deepen the twist slightly, enhancing the stretch and its benefits on the spine and abdominal area.

5. To switch sides, gently release the twist and turn to face the right side of the chair. Repeat the twisting motion on this side to ensure a balanced, symmetrical stretch.

This chapter has focused on enhancing flexibility and mobility through specific chair yoga exercises. By incorporating these movements into your routine, you can significantly improve your range of motion and ease of movement. Improved flexibility and mobility are essential for performing daily tasks with greater ease and confidence, reducing the risk of injury, and enhancing overall physical health.

Regular practice of these chair yoga exercises will help you enjoy a more active and fulfilling lifestyle, empowering you to move with increased confidence and physical capability. Whether it's reaching, bending, or walking, enhanced flexibility and mobility contribute to a more independent and enjoyable daily life.

CHAPTER 7
CHAIR YOGA FOR POSTURE AND ALIGNMENT

Good posture and proper alignment are vital for overall health and well-being, particularly as we age. Poor posture can lead to various issues, such as back pain, reduced mobility, and a higher risk of falls. By incorporating exercises that improve posture and alignment, we can enhance balance, stability, and overall body mechanics.

This chapter will explore a variety of chair yoga poses designed to promote better posture and alignment. These exercises are accessible for seniors and aim to strengthen the muscles that support proper alignment, reduce tension, and increase body awareness. Enhanced posture and alignment contribute to greater ease in daily activities, increased confidence, and a reduced risk of injury.

Good posture is more than just standing up straight; it involves maintaining the natural curves of your spine and ensuring that your body is properly aligned. Proper alignment helps distribute your weight evenly, reducing strain on your muscles and joints.

Consider how often you sit, stand, or move throughout the day. Your posture and alignment play a significant role in these activities:

» **Sitting and Standing**: Maintaining proper posture ensures that you sit and stand with ease, reducing the risk of back and neck pain.

» **Moving and Walking**: Good alignment supports better balance and stability, making it easier to walk and move without discomfort.

» **Performing Daily Tasks**: Proper posture and alignment make everyday activities, like reaching, bending, and lifting, safer and more efficient.

By focusing on your posture and alignment, you can perform these tasks more comfortably and confidently, enhancing your overall quality of life.

POSTURE AND ALIGNMENT POSES

Seated Mountain Pose

Helps with:	
» **Improved posture** This pose encourages proper spinal alignment, promoting better posture.	» **Muscle strengthening** Engaging the core and back muscles helps build strength in these areas.
» **Improved balance and coordination** Maintaining a strong and steady position enhances overall stability and coordination.	
Safety Precautions:	
- Use the back of the chair for support if needed to help maintain balance and stability. - Keep your core muscles engaged to support your spine.	

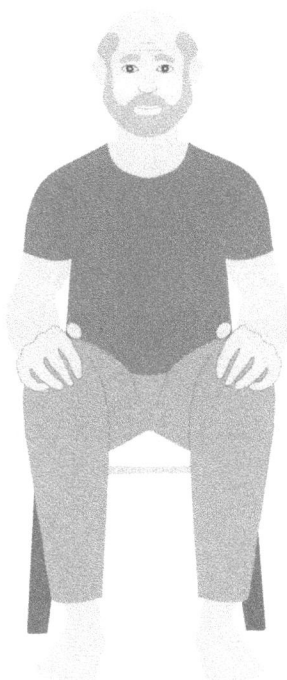

1. Sit comfortably on a sturdy chair with your feet flat on the ground, hip-width apart. Ensure your back is straight, and your shoulders are relaxed.

2. Place your hands on your thighs or let them rest by your sides. Engage your core muscles to support your spine.

3. Inhale deeply and lengthen your spine, imagining a string pulling the top of your head towards the ceiling. Sit up tall, elongating your neck and keeping your chin parallel to the floor.

4. Roll your shoulders back and down, opening your chest and maintaining a relaxed posture.

5. Press your feet firmly into the ground, feeling the connection with the floor. Lightly engage your thigh muscles to stabilize your lower body.

6. Hold the position for several breaths, focusing on maintaining alignment and length in your spine. Breathe deeply and steadily.

7. After holding the pose for a few breaths, release the engagement in your muscles and relax.

Seated Fish Pose

Helps with:	
» **Pain reduction** This pose stretches the chest, neck, and upper back, helping to alleviate pain and discomfort in these areas.	» **Reduced muscle tension** Stretching the chest and shoulder muscles helps release tightness and reduce muscle tension, promoting relaxation.
» **Improved posture** By opening the chest and aligning the spine, this pose encourages proper posture and reduces the risk of slouching.	» **Enhanced joint flexibility** Increases flexibility in the shoulders, chest, and upper back, improving overall mobility.
Safety Precautions: - Ensure your chair is stable and will not slide. - Be mindful to lift the chest and open the shoulders without straining the neck. - If you experience any discomfort in your lower back, adjust your hand placement or reduce the backbend.	

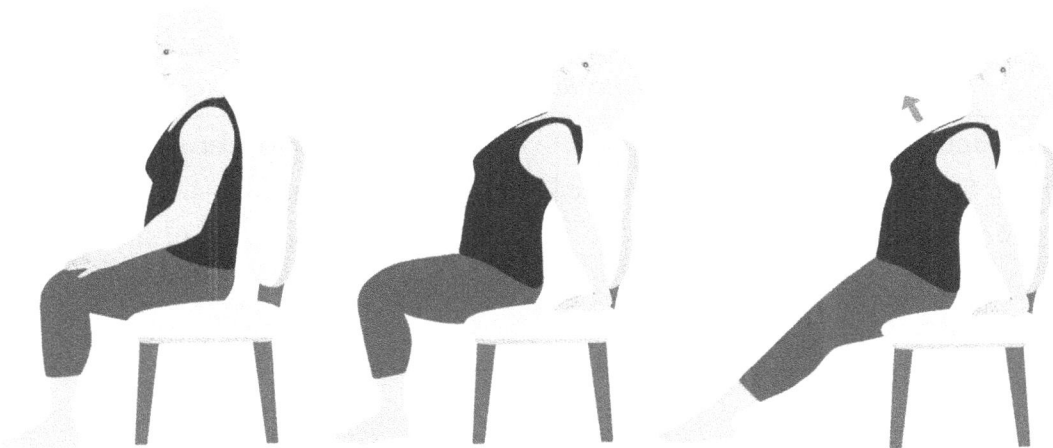

Steps:

1. Begin in a seated mountain pose, sitting upright with your feet pressed firmly into the floor and your spine lengthened.

2. Place your hands on your hips, lower back, or with fingertips on the seat of the chair behind you, fingers pointing forward, depending on what feels most comfortable and supportive.

3. Draw your shoulder blades toward each other, lifting your sternum to open the chest.

4. You may keep your feet in the sitting mountain position or extend your legs, pressing into the bottom of your feet and engaging your thighs for added stability and stretch.

5. Lift your chin slightly, directing your gaze towards the seam where the roof meets the wall, creating a gentle extension in the neck.

6. If comfortable, lean back slightly and press into your palms or the seat of the chair to deepen the chest expansion. Ensure this movement is gradual and controlled to avoid straining the back.

7. Optionally, you can extend your lower jaw forward and smile gently. This action activates the throat and front of the neck, enhancing the stretch without compressing the back of the neck.

8. Breathe deeply into the front of your torso, allowing the breath to facilitate a deeper opening in the chest and shoulders.

9. To come out of the pose, slowly lift your torso back to an upright seated position. Sit quietly for a breath or two, allowing your body to integrate the effects of the pose.

Seated Shoulder Shrugs

Helps with:	
» **Reduced muscle tension** This exercise helps release tightness in the shoulders and neck.	» **Improved circulation** The up-and-down movement promotes blood flow to the shoulder and neck area.
» **Pain reduction** Regular shoulder shrugs can help alleviate tension-related pain in the shoulders and neck.	

Safety Precautions:
- Move slowly and avoid overexerting the shoulder muscles.

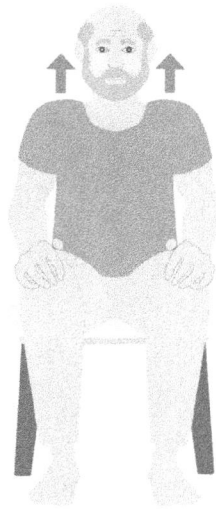

Steps:

1. Sit upright in a chair with your feet firmly planted on the floor. This stable base supports proper posture and alignment throughout the exercise.

2. Inhale deeply, and with intention, lift your shoulders towards your ears. This upward movement should be controlled, engaging the muscles without straining them.

3. As you exhale, consciously release your shoulders back down. This downward motion encourages relaxation and the release of any built-up tension.

4. Repeat the shrugging motion 5-10 times, focusing on smooth, deliberate movements. Each shrug should contribute to a greater sense of ease in your shoulders and neck.

Seated Forward Fold

Helps with:	
» **Enhanced joint flexibility** This pose stretches the spine, hips, and hamstrings, improving overall flexibility.	» **Pain reduction** It helps to relieve lower back pain by stretching and lengthening the spine.
» **Improved circulation** Forward bending increases blood flow to the spine and pelvic region.	» **Better muscle elasticity** Regular practice improves the elasticity of the muscles and connective tissues.

Safety Precautions:

- Bend from your hips, not your waist. Start the movement at your hip joint, where your thigh meets your pelvis.
- Avoid if you have severe lower back issues.

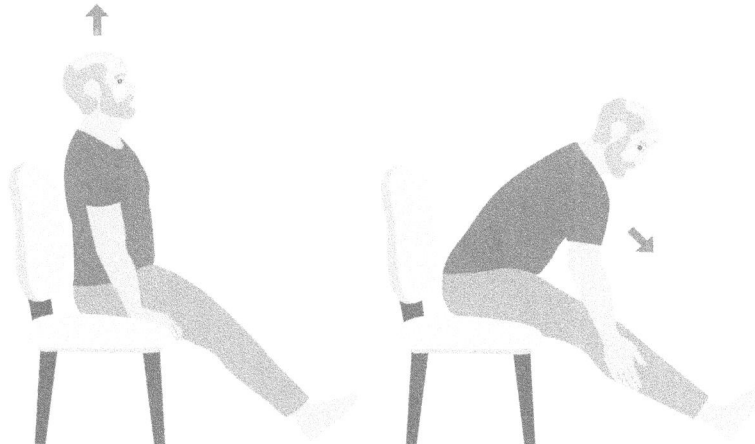

Steps:

1. Begin by sitting upright, legs extended before you, with feet positioned hip-width apart. Let this be your foundation of stability and balance.

2. Inhale deeply, inviting length into your spine, envisioning each vertebra stretching towards the sky.

3. On your exhale, pivot gracefully from your hips (to bend from the hips push your hips back while keeping your spine long and chest open), folding forward as if reaching for a moment of tranquility. Extend your hands towards your feet, embodying the gentle embrace of calm.

4. Hold this forward embrace for several nurturing breaths, allowing tension to melt away with each exhale.

5. To conclude, slowly ascend back to an upright position, carrying with you the peace and stretch you've cultivated.

Chair Warrior I Variation

Helps with:	
» **Muscle strengthening** This pose strengthens the legs, hips, and core, building overall lower body strength.	» **Improved balance and coordination** The warrior stance enhances stability and coordination.

» **Improved posture**
Engaging the core and maintaining proper alignment helps improve overall posture.

Safety Precautions:

- Ensure the chair is stable and doesn't slide.
- Avoid overstraining the back leg.

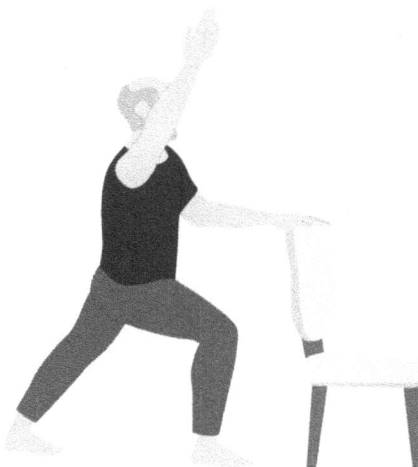

Steps:

1. Begin by standing behind a chair, using the back of the chair for support. This ensures stability and safety throughout the exercise.

2. Step your right foot forward, bending the knee to create a lunge position. Ensure your left leg remains straight with the heel firmly planted on the ground, providing a stretch through the back leg.

3. As you find your balance, lift your arms overhead. You can choose to join your palms for added stretch through the upper body or keep them shoulder-width apart if that's more comfortable.

4. Focus your gaze straight ahead or slightly upwards, aligning your posture and deepening the stretch across your chest and hips. Hold this position for a few deep breaths, allowing your body to settle into the pose.

5. Gently release the pose, returning to your starting position, and then switch legs, repeating the steps with your left leg forward.

Seated Warrior II Arms

Helps with:	
» **Muscle strengthening** Engages and strengthens the shoulders, arms, and upper back muscles.	» **Improved balance and coordination** Holding the arms extended helps enhance overall stability and coordination.
» **Enhanced joint flexibility** Increases flexibility in the shoulders and upper back.	» **Improved posture** Encourages proper spinal alignment and shoulder positioning, promoting better overall posture.
Safety Precautions:	
- Keep the shoulder blades down and back to avoid tension	

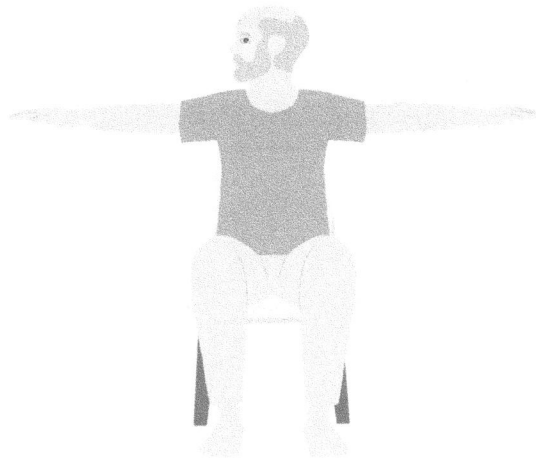

Steps:

1. Begin by sitting upright in a chair, ensuring your feet are flat on the ground. This stable base aids in maintaining proper posture throughout the exercise.

2. Stretch your arms out to either side, reaching them to shoulder height with your palms facing down. This action engages the muscles in your arms and shoulders, promoting strength and flexibility.

3. Turn your head to gaze over your right hand, extending the stretch and enhancing your focus. This not only helps in stretching the neck muscles but also aids in concentration and mental clarity.

4. Hold this position for several deep breaths, encouraging a deeper engagement with each exhale. Ensure your shoulder blades are drawn down and back to prevent any unnecessary tension in your neck and shoulders.

5. Gently bring your gaze back to the center before turning to look over your left hand, effectively repeating the pose on this side. This ensures a balanced stretch and strength enhancement across both sides of your body.

Seated Neck Roll and Stretch

Helps with:	
» **Pain reduction** This stretch relieves tension in the neck, reducing pain and discomfort.	» **Reduced muscle tension** Gently rolling and stretching the neck muscles helps release tightness and reduce muscle tension.
» **Improved posture** Regular practice can help correct forward head posture and improve overall neck alignment.	
Safety Precautions:	
- Perform movements gently to avoid strain. - If you experience dizziness, pause and return to a neutral position.	

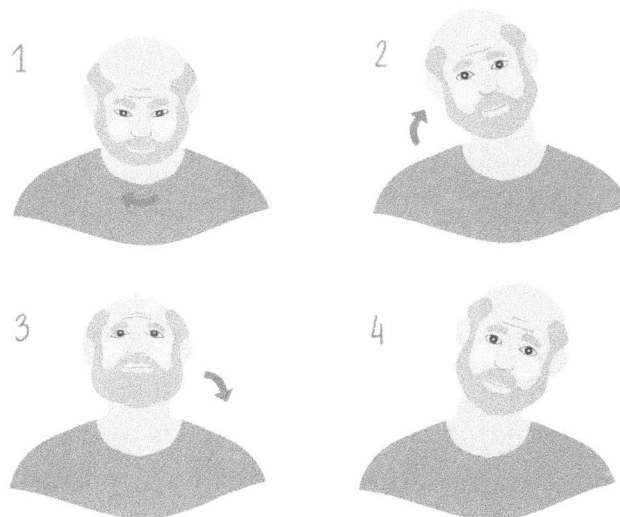

Steps:

1. Begin by sitting in a comfortable chair with your spine aligned and upright. This posture ensures a safe foundation for the exercise.

2. Slowly tilt your head forward, guiding your chin towards your chest. This initial movement starts the stretch and begins to release tension in the neck.

3. Gently roll your head to the right, aiming to bring your ear closer to your shoulder. This action stretches the side neck muscles, aiding in flexibility.

4. Continue the motion by rolling your head backward and then to the left, completing a smooth, circular movement. This sequence helps to evenly distribute the stretch across the neck muscles.

5. Perform 3-5 rolls in each direction, moving at a pace that feels comfortable and safe. Ensure each roll is performed gently to avoid any strain.

Incorporating these chair yoga exercises into your daily routine will significantly improve your posture and alignment. Good posture not only reduces pain but also enhances balance and overall mobility, contributing to a more active and fulfilling lifestyle.

Imagine moving through your day with improved posture: less back pain, easier performance of daily tasks, and increased confidence in your movements. By practicing these exercises regularly, you take proactive steps to improve your physical health and maintain your independence.

Enhancing your posture and alignment also means reducing tension in your muscles and joints, leading to a more relaxed and comfortable body. With consistent practice, you will develop the muscle strength and body awareness needed to maintain good posture throughout the day.

These chair yoga exercises are designed to be gentle yet effective, ensuring you can safely improve your posture and alignment. Regular practice will help you enjoy a more active, independent, and confident daily life. Embrace these movements and experience the positive changes in your body mechanics and overall well-being. Keep practicing and enjoy the benefits of better posture and alignment. You've got this!

CHAPTER 8
YOUR FLEXIBLE CHAIR YOGA ROUTINE FOR STRENGTH

To help you get started, here is a sample weekly routine plan. This plan is designed to be flexible, allowing you to easily adjust and change the exercises based on which areas you want to focus.

Instructions:

1. **Begin each day with a breathing technique and some warm-up exercises.** This will help to center your mind and prepare your body for the chair yoga session.

2. **Follow the sequence of poses as outlined for each day.** Hold each pose for 30 - 45 seconds based on how you feel.

3. **Take a short pause of 15 seconds between each exercise or pose.** Use this time to breathe normally and prepare for the next pose.

4. **Remember to go at your own pace.** It's important to listen to your body and not push beyond comfort. If you experience any discomfort, modify the pose or skip it as needed.

5. **Begin with the goal of practicing these chair yoga workouts daily.** I know that you're busy, but I've found that this consistent approach helps students to establish a routine and maximize the benefits of the program.
    » However, it's important to listen to your body and be mindful of your energy levels and physical comfort.
    » If you find that daily practice is too demanding, or if you experience any discomfort, it's perfectly fine to adjust your schedule.
    » In such cases, aim to complete the workouts 4 to 5 times a week instead.
    » This adjustment ensures that you still maintain regular practice while giving your body adequate time to rest and recover.

I'm here to support you on your journey to a healthier, happier life. If you have any questions, concerns, or would like a few words of encouragement, please don't hesitate to reach out (jcharrisonbooks@gmail.com).

Here is an example of what doing some exercises from Part III - chapter 3 might look like.

WEEK 1 SAMPLE ROUTINE FOR STRENGTH

Box Breathing (perform for 30-45s, page 22)

INHALE 4 SECONDS   HOLD 4 SECONDS   EXHALE 4 SECONDS   HOLD 4 SECONDS

Ankle and Wrist Rotations (30-45s, page 31)	Torso Twists (30-45s, page 30)	Seated Arm Circles (30-45s, page 171)
Seated Chest Opener (30-45s, page 172)	Seated Arm Swings (30-45s, page 175)	Seated Goddess Pose (30-45s, page 176)

Remember to take a short pause of 15 seconds between each exercise or pose.

For week 2 feel free to try some of the other exercises from Chapter 3 or you can do exercises from a different chapter to target another area in your body.

CONCLUSION

As we come to the end of this journey through chair yoga for building strength, let's take a moment to reflect on the progress you've made and the tools you've gained to enhance your well-being. Chair yoga is a powerful method to improve strength, mobility, and overall health, especially for seniors. We've explored various aspects of physical health and provided exercises to target different areas of your body.

First, we focused on strengthening your core, a crucial component for overall stability and balance. By engaging in exercises that target your abdominal and back muscles, you can maintain better posture and reduce the risk of falls. Then, we moved on to building upper body strength, emphasizing the importance of strong arms, shoulders, and chest. These exercises are designed to make daily tasks like lifting and carrying items easier and safer for you.

In our exploration of lower body strength, we highlighted the significance of strong legs and hips for mobility and balance. The targeted exercises you learned help improve your ability to walk, climb stairs, and stand up from a seated position with greater ease. We also delved into enhancing your balance and coordination, providing exercises to reduce the risk of falls and promote safer, more confident movements.

Flexibility and mobility are vital for performing everyday activities with ease. By incorporating exercises that reduce stiffness and improve your range of motion, you can make daily movements smoother and more comfortable. Lastly, we focused on maintaining proper posture and alignment to prevent pain and improve overall body mechanics. These exercises strengthen the muscles that support good posture, helping you move more comfortably and confidently.

Each chapter offered you valuable exercises to strengthen different aspects of your body, contributing to a comprehensive approach to your physical health. But the journey doesn't end here.

It's essential to continue incorporating chair yoga into your daily routine to fully reap its long-term benefits. Regular practice will lead to enhanced strength, better balance, reduced pain, and an improved quality of life. Remember, consistency is key. By dedicating time each day to these exercises, you are investing in your health and independence.

Setting personal goals can keep you motivated and help you track your progress. Whether your aim is to increase flexibility, improve balance, or build strength, having clear objectives will keep you focused. Start with realistic, achievable goals and monitor your progress over time. Celebrate every milestone, no matter how small, and use your achievements as motivation to keep going.

Adopting a holistic approach to health and aging is vital. Chair yoga is most effective when combined with other healthy habits. Ensure you eat a balanced diet, get adequate rest, and incorporate mental relaxation techniques into your routine. This comprehensive approach will help you achieve optimal health and well-being.

As we conclude, remember that it's never too late to start improving your health and well-being. By choosing to practice chair yoga, you've taken a significant step towards a healthier, stronger, and more fulfilling life. Keep practicing, stay consistent, and embrace the journey towards better health.

Thank you for committing to this journey with chair yoga. Your dedication to your well-being is truly inspiring. You've got this, and we're cheering you on every step of the way.

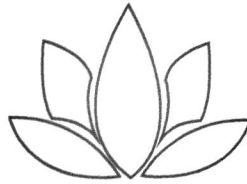

REFERENCES

Bao, W., Sun, Y., Zhang, T., Zou, L., Wu, X., Wang, D., & Chen, Z. (2020). Exercise Programs for Muscle Mass, Muscle Strength and Physical Performance in Older Adults with Sarcopenia: A Systematic Review and Meta-Analysis. Aging and Disease, 11, 863 - 873. https://doi.org/10.14336/ad.2019.1012.

Bonura, K., & Tenenbaum, G. (2014). Effects of yoga on psychological health in older adults. Journal of physical activity & health, 11 7, 1334-41. https://doi.org/10.1123/jpah.2012-0365.

Fishman, L. (2021). Yoga and Bone Health. Orthopaedic Nursing, 40, 169 - 179. https://doi.org/10.1097/NOR.0000000000000757.

Ghahramani, A. (2014). The effect of the relaxation training on the general health and selected physical fitness factors affecting seniors balance. Asian journal of multidisciplinary studies, 3.

Law, S., Leung, A., & Xu, C. (2021). Is Yoga possible for elderly care? Geriatric Care. https://doi.org/10.4081/GC.2021.9815.

Marciniak, R., Sheardová, K., Čermaková, P., Hudeček, D., Šumec, R., & Hort, J. (2014). Effect of Meditation on Cognitive Functions in Context of Aging and Neurodegenerative Diseases. Frontiers in Behavioral Neuroscience, 8. https://doi.org/10.3389/fnbeh.2014.00017.

McArthur, C., Laprade, J., & Giangregorio, L. (2016). Suggestions for Adapting Yoga to the Needs of Older Adults with Osteoporosis.. Journal of alternative and complementary medicine, 22 3, 223-6. https://doi.org/10.1089/acm.2014.0397.

McCaffrey, R., Park, J., Newman, D., & Hagen, D. (2014). The effect of chair yoga in older adults with moderate and severe Alzheimer's disease. Research in gerontological nursing, 7 4, 171-7. https://doi.org/10.3928/19404921-20140218-01.

Park, J., & McCaffrey, R. (2012). Chair yoga: benefits for community-dwelling older adults with osteoarthritis. Journal of gerontological nursing, 38 5, 12-22; quiz 24-5. https://doi.org/10.3928/00989134-20120410-01.

Park, J., Newman, D., McCaffrey, R., Garrido, J., Riccio, M., & Liehr, P. (2016). The Effect of Chair Yoga on Biopsychosocial Changes in English- and Spanish-Speaking Community-Dwelling Older Adults with Lower-Extremity Osteoarthritis. Journal of Gerontological Social Work, 59, 604 - 626. https://doi.org/10.1080/01634372.2016.1239234.

Park, J., Tolea, M., Rosenfeld, A., Arcay, V., Karson, J., Lopes, Y., Small, K., & Galvin, J. (2018). FEASIBILITY AND EFFECTS OF CHAIR YOGA TO MANAGE DEMENTIA SYMPTOMS IN OLDER ADULTS. Innovation in Aging. https://doi.org/10.1093/GERONI/IGY023.1142.

Yao, C., & Tseng, C. (2019). Effectiveness of Chair Yoga for Improving the Functional Fitness and Well-being of Female Community-Dwelling Older Adults With Low Physical Activities. Topics in Geriatric Rehabilitation, 35, 248 - 254. https://doi.org/10.1097/TGR.0000000000000242.

You, S., Hong, S., & Moon, K. (2013). Effects of Hatha Yoga Practice on the Elderly Having Chronic Back Pain Because of Computer Usage. The Journal of the Korea institute of electronic communication sciences, 8, 1121-1128. https://doi.org/10.13067/JKIECS.2013.8.7.1121.

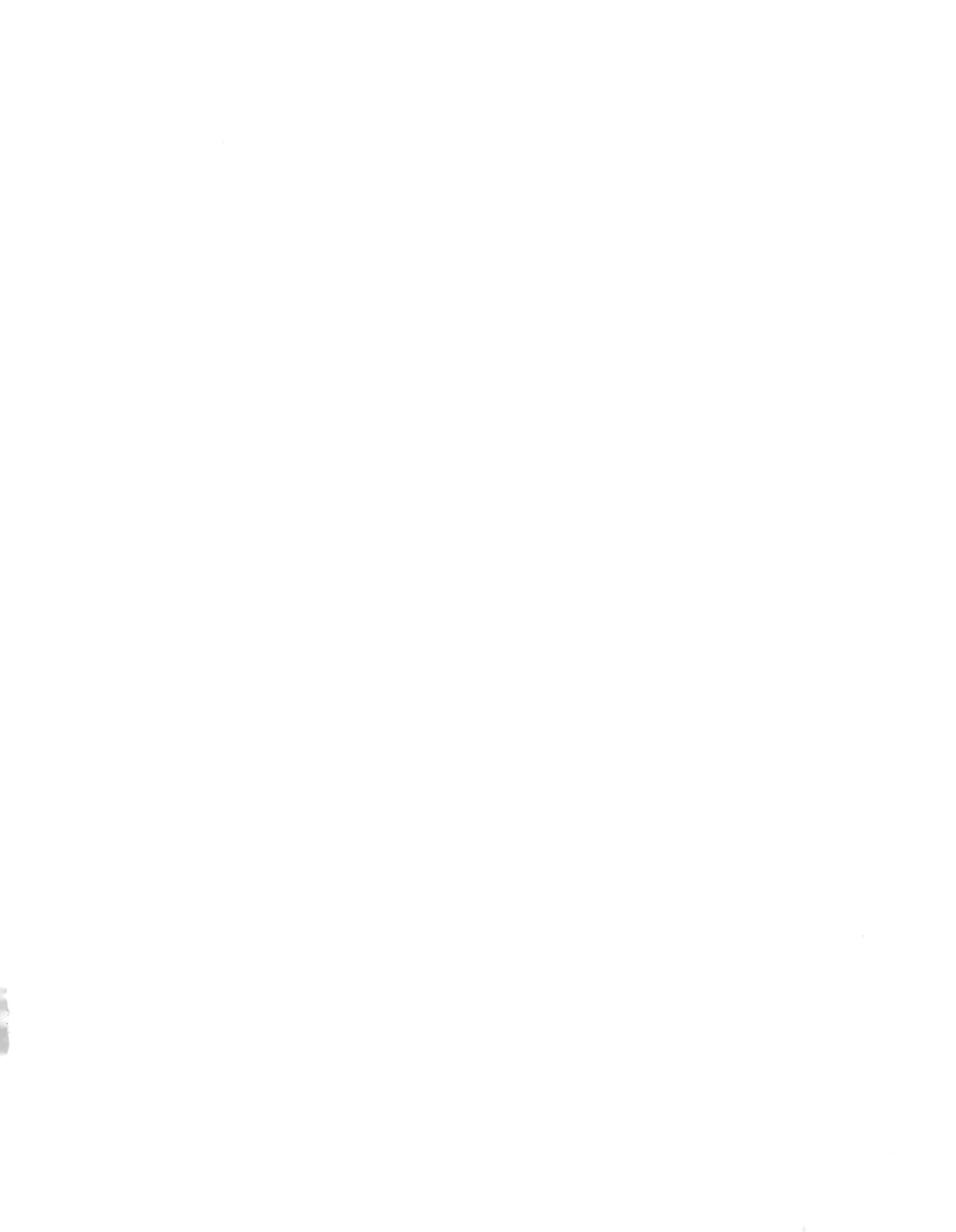